Palgrave Texts in Counselling and Psychotherapy

Series Editors
Arlene Vetere
Family Therapy and Systemic Practice
VID Specialized University
Oslo, Norway

Rudi Dallos
Clinical Psychology
Plymouth University
Plymouth, UK

This series introduces readers to the theory and practice of counselling and psychotherapy across a wide range of topical issues. Ideal for both trainees and practitioners, the books will appeal to anyone wishing to use counselling and psychotherapeutic skills and will be particularly relevant to workers in health, education, social work and related settings. The books in this series emphasise an integrative orientation weaving together a variety of models including, psychodynamic, attachment, trauma, narrative and systemic ideas. The books are written in an accessible and readable style with a focus on practice. Each text offers theoretical background and guidance for practice, with creative use of clinical examples.

Arlene Vetere, Professor of Family Therapy and Systemic Practice at VID Specialized University, Oslo, Norway.

Rudi Dallos, Emeritus Professor, Dept. of Clinical Psychology, University of Plymouth, UK.

Michelle O'Reilly • Nikki Kiyimba

Communicating With Families

Taking The Language of Mental Health From Research to Practice

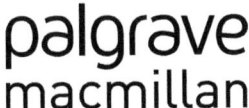

Michelle O'Reilly
Media, Communication and Sociology
University of Leicester, and
FYPC-LD-A, Leicestershire Partnership
NHS Trust
Leicester, UK

Nikki Kiyimba
Mātai Rongo Psychological Services
Tauranga, New Zealand

ISSN 2662-9127   ISSN 2662-9135 (electronic)
Palgrave Texts in Counselling and Psychotherapy
ISBN 978-3-031-30417-0   ISBN 978-3-031-30418-7 (eBook)
https://doi.org/10.1007/978-3-031-30418-7

© Springer Nature Switzerland AG 2023

This work is subject to copyright. All rights are solely and exclusively licensed by the Publisher, whether the whole or part of the material is concerned, specifically the rights of translation, reprinting, reuse of illustrations, recitation, broadcasting, reproduction on microfilms or in any other physical way, and transmission or information storage and retrieval, electronic adaptation, computer software, or by similar or dissimilar methodology now known or hereafter developed.

The use of general descriptive names, registered names, trademarks, service marks, etc. in this publication does not imply, even in the absence of a specific statement, that such names are exempt from the relevant protective laws and regulations and therefore free for general use.

The publisher, the authors, and the editors are safe to assume that the advice and information in this book are believed to be true and accurate at the date of publication. Neither the publisher nor the authors or the editors give a warranty, expressed or implied, with respect to the material contained herein or for any errors or omissions that may have been made. The publisher remains neutral with regard to jurisdictional claims in published maps and institutional affiliations.

This Palgrave Macmillan imprint is published by the registered company Springer Nature Switzerland AG.
The registered company address is: Gewerbestrasse 11, 6330 Cham, Switzerland

Foreword

Central to how family therapists and other professionals practice when working with families, is the art of conversation. However, typically the problems experienced by families and practitioners' responses to them are accounted for in practitioners' terms associated with their preferred theories and models of practice. Conversations within families, like those between family members and therapists, in other words, tend to exemplify the beliefs and modes of intervention adopted by therapist-authors. When research evidence is used to support these beliefs and modes of interventions, it focuses on outcomes (e.g., client satisfaction, symptom checklists) but not on what actually occurs in the conversational work with families in their everyday institutional settings.

Michelle O'Reilly and Nikki Kiyimba draw on their considerable research of mental health communications, to focus on the conversational work in mental health practice with families. Family life and mental health interactions, like family therapy, mental health assessments, and family social work are sites where different social realities are constructed through talking. Using detailed analyses of actual therapy and other mental health setting interactions, O'Reilly and Kiyimba zoom in to provide valuable ways of making sense of how family members and practitioners talk across wide-ranging aspects of family mental health practice and therapy. They do this by bringing readers *inside* relevant junctures in the conversations of therapy, to show how the challenging practice of work with families is accomplished, turn by conversational turn. After reviewing how conversational interactions construct family life in normal and problematic ways, they turn to topics such as practitioners forming and maintaining good relations with families and family members, engaging children's participation and competence in institutional interactions, managing sensitive topics with children present, avoiding shame and blame, talking about risks within families, and using video recordings of practice as learning and supervision resources for family practitioners. Transcripts used in elaborating these topics show not only what was said in these interactions but bring out important dimensions of how talk was performed and received in the immediacies of therapy's conversational turn-taking. Literally, readers are shown how therapeutic developments are co-constructed through how family members and practitioners use their words and ways of talking together.

O'Reilly and Kiyimba have crystallised years of painstaking microanalysis of how mental health professionals and service users talk with each other to zero in on daunting but key aspects of successful practices like family therapy and mental health assessments. They draw from striking examples of actual talk to show how the conversational work with families gets done in ways that can newly sensitise as well as enhance skilled professional interactions. This is a clearly written and highly practical book that will be welcomed by students of therapy and other related mental health disciplines, as well as skilled practitioners.

University of Calgary Tom Strong
Calgary, AB, Canada

Tom Strong is a professor and counsellor-educator who recently retired from the University of Calgary. He writes on the collaborative, critical, and practical potentials of discursive approaches to psychotherapy—most recently on concept critique and development (particularly with respect to therapy and research), and critical mental health. Among Tom's books are *Medicalizing Counselling: Issues and Tensions*; *Patterns in Interpersonal Interactions* (co-edited with Karl Tomm, Sally St. George, and Dan Wulff); and *Social Constructionism: Sources and Stirrings in Theory and Practice* (co-authored with Andy Lock), and he is co-editing (with Olga Smoliak, Eleftheria Tseliou, Saliha Bava, and Peter Muntigl) the *Routledge International Handbook of Postmodern Therapies*. For Tom's website and contact details, please see: https://wpsites.ucalgary.ca/tom-strong/.

Acknowledgements

Michelle and Nikki would like to extend a very large thank you to Professor Tom Strong for taking the time to review the whole book for us and for providing the interesting foreword. Tom provided some helpful and practical feedback from an academic and clinical perspective and our book is much stronger for it.

We are also grateful to all the clinical practitioners who contributed a reflective box for each of the chapters. These practitioners also took the time to comment on the chapter they contributed to and helped to shape the direction of that chapter. In order of their contribution, therefore, we thank, Clement Chihota, Philip Archard, Michelle Youngs, Sadiyya Haffejee, Olga Smoliak, Jenny Phaure, Erin O'Neill, and Alison Drewett.

We extend thanks to the team at Palgrave for their support in producing this manuscript, and to the editors of the series for the invitation, Rudi Dallos and Arlene Vetere.

Finally, and importantly, we are very appreciative of all the participants, families, and clinical practitioners, who consented to be part of the different research projects that are drawn upon throughout the book. We are also grateful for the ongoing support of our partners and families that has allowed us to make the completion of this book possible.

Contents

Part I Theoretical Context   1

1 Systems Within Systems: Families in Society   3
    Introduction   3
    Language and Communication   4
    Stigma   7
    Pathology   9
    Social Meta-Narratives   11
    Research Data   16
    Author Positionality   22
    Final Thoughts   24
    References   25

2 Family Dynamics and Constructs   29
    Introduction   29
    What Constitutes the Family?   30
    Vulnerability and Resilience Factors in the Family   36
    Working with Families in Mental Health   44
    Final Thoughts   46
    References   49

3	**Forming and Maintaining Good Relationships**	53
	Introduction	53
	The Therapeutic Relationship	54
	Rupture	61
	Interruptions	69
	Final Thoughts	77
	References	80
Part II	**Engaging Children**	**85**
4	**Designing Questions with Children**	87
	Introduction	87
	The Value of Questions and the Importance of Question Design	88
	Different Ways of Using Questions	89
	'Why Are You Here?' Questions	96
	Using Why Questions	99
	The Miracle Question	102
	You Said Prefaced Questions	106
	Circular Questions	108
	Final Thoughts	111
	References	113
5	**Using Creative Activities with Children**	117
	Introduction	117
	Subjective Units of Distress	118
	Stress Bucket	121
	Using Symbols and Archetypes	124
	A Shift to Digital	136
	Final Thoughts	141
	References	144
6	**Children's Competence**	147
	Introduction	147
	Situated Interactional Competence	149

Competence to Report One's Own Motivations, Feelings and Thoughts	158
Knowledge of the Feelings and Thoughts of Others	161
Final Thoughts	168
References	171

Part III   Attending to the Different Needs of Family Members   173

7   Managing Age-Appropriate Conversations with Children Present   175

Introduction	175
Appropriate Topics of Conversation	176
Talking About the Child, with the Child Present	180
Negotiating Time with Parents and Children Separately	184
Final Thoughts	192
References	195

8   Avoiding Shame and Blame   197

Introduction	197
Identity Construction and the Role of the Good Parent	200
Parent Blaming	203
Managing Responsibility and Blame	206
Final Thoughts	211
References	214

9   How to Talk About Risk   217

Introduction	217
How to Have a Conversation About Risk	220
Safeguarding	239
Responsibility and Boundaries	244
Final Thoughts	245
References	248

10	**Using Naturally Occurring Data for Professional Development**	253
	Introduction	253
	Using Recordings of Naturally Occurring Activities	254
	Using Naturally Occurring Text-Based Documents	259
	Using Naturally Occurring Data for Supervision	261
	Using Reflective Interventionist Conversation Analysis (RICA)	265
	Final Thoughts	267
	References	268

Appendix: Jefferson Transcription – Overview of Symbols Used 271

Index 273

About the Authors

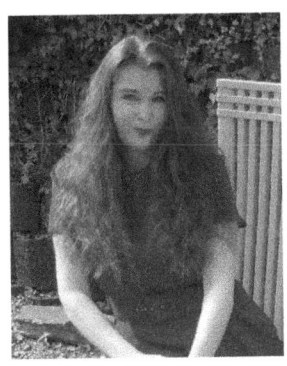

Michelle O'Reilly, BSc [hons], MSc, MA, PhD is Associate Professor of Communication in Mental Health at the University of Leicester and a Research Consultant and Quality Improvement Advisor for Leicestershire Partnership NHS Trust. Michelle is also a Chartered Psychologist in Health. Michelle has research interests in mental health and social media, self-harm and suicidal behaviour, neurodevelopmental conditions, and child mental health services, such as mental health assessments and family therapy. Michelle recently won the Anselm Strauss Award for Qualitative Family Research for her co-authored contribution on discursive psychology in this area (with Nikki Kiyimba and Jessica Lester). Michelle has expertise in qualitative methodologies and specialises in discursive psychology and conversation analysis. Michelle has written considerably in the field of research methods and has written practical guidance for clinical practitioners on how to do qualitative research.

About the Authors

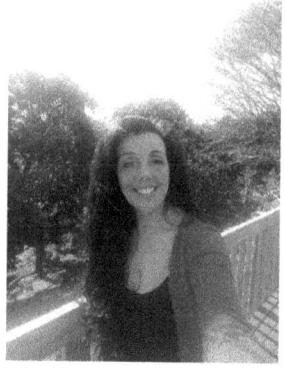

Nikki Kiyimba, BSc [Hons], PhD, DClinPsy is a clinical academic and Chartered Consultant Clinical Psychologist. Nikki has extensive experience in tertiary education, and of programme leadership for two Masters' and a taught Doctorate in the UK. She is an ongoing editorial member for the journal *Crisis, Illness and Loss* and guest editor and peer reviewer for several other international journals. She has co-authored three textbooks on research methods and an extensive publication history at the intersection of the fields of mental health, spirituality, trauma, and discursive practice. Having developed Aotearoa, New Zealand's first Postgraduate Certificate in Responding to Trauma, she is now Clinical Director of Mātai Rongo, based in the beautiful Bay of Plenty. Mātai Rongo is a specialist Trauma-informed psychology service providing training, supervision, and consultancy as well as trauma-responsive clinical work with families and individuals.

Abbreviations

ACEs	Adverse childhood experiences
CA	Conversation analysis
CAMHS	Child and adolescent mental health services
CPN	Community psychiatric nurse
DA	Discourse analysis
DP	Discursive psychology
DSM	Diagnostic and statistical manual of mental disorders
ECF	Extreme case formulation
FT	Family therapist
GMC	General Medical Council
ICD	International classification of diseases
IPV	Intimate partner violence
MHN	Mental health nurse (see CPN)
NHS	National Health Service
NT	Narrative Therapy
OCD	Obsessive compulsive disorder
RICA	Reflective interventionist conversation analysis
SUDs	Subjective units of distress
TRP	Transition relevance place
UNCRC	United Nations Convention on the Rights of the Child

List of Figures

Fig. 2.1	Stress vulnerability model	41
Fig. 2.2	Transactional model of stress	42
Fig. 5.1	Bucket sizes. (Illustrations taken from Kiyimba, 2020)	122
Fig. 5.2	Adverse events (taken from Kiyimba, 2020)	122
Fig. 5.3	Releasing the pressure	123
Fig. 5.4	The dialectical balance	128
Fig. 6.1	K+-K− knowledge continuum in relation to institutional knowledge	156
Fig. 6.2	The knowledge continuum reversed	159

List of Tables

Table 2.1	The five P's	40
Table 2.2	Overview of ACEs	43
Table 3.1	DeAngelis (2019) findings from 16 meta-analyses on therapeutic relationships	55
Table 4.1	The sequence	107
Table 8.1	Different kinds of stigma (Clement et al., 2015)	203

List of Boxes

Box 1.1	Activity on Language	21
Box 1.2	Key Points	25
Box 2.1	Reflective Activity on Childhood	35
Box 2.2	Reflective Activity on the Transactional Model of Stress	42
Box 2.3	Practitioner Voice, Clement Chihota	47
Box 2.4	Key Points	48
Box 3.1	Reflective Activity on Rupture	69
Box 3.2	Practitioner Voice, Philip Archard	78
Box 3.3	Key Points	80
Box 4.1	Alternative Framings	101
Box 4.2	Reflective Activity on Using Why Questions	102
Box 4.3	Reflective Activity on the Miracle Question	106
Box 4.4	Practitioner Voice, Michelle Youngs	111
Box 4.5	Key Points	113
Box 5.1	Reflective Activity on Creative Techniques	124
Box 5.2	Reflective Activity on Using Symbols	131
Box 5.3	Reflective Activity on Creative Activities Online	139
Box 5.4	Reflective Activity on the Dialectical Balance in Online Work	140
Box 5.5	Practitioner Voice, Sadiyya Haffejee	142
Box 5.6	Key Points	143
Box 6.1	Reflective Activity on Preparations	155
Box 6.2	Reflective Activity on Access to Knowledge of Other People	162
Box 6.3	Practitioner Voice, Olga Smoliak	168

Box 6.4	Key Points	170
Box 7.1	Reflective activity on Types of Conversations	180
Box 7.2	Reflective Activity on Using the Tools in Your Practice	184
Box 7.3	Practitioner Voice, Jenny Phaure	193
Box 7.4	Key Points About Managing Togetherness and Separateness in Family Conversations	194
Box 8.1	Reflective Activity: Noticing Dichotomous Accounting Practices	200
Box 8.2	Reflective Activity: Overcoming Barriers to Help-Seeking	205
Box 8.3	Practitioner Voice, Erin O'Neill	212
Box 8.4	Key Points	213
Box 9.1	Reflective Activity on Questions About Risk	226
Box 9.2	Reflective Activity on IPV and Child Abuse Questions (Hornor, 2005, p. 209)	234
Box 9.3	Reflecting on the Personal Impact of Working with Risk	245
Box 9.4	Practitioner Voice, Alison Drewett	246
Box 9.5	Key Points	248

Part I

Theoretical Context

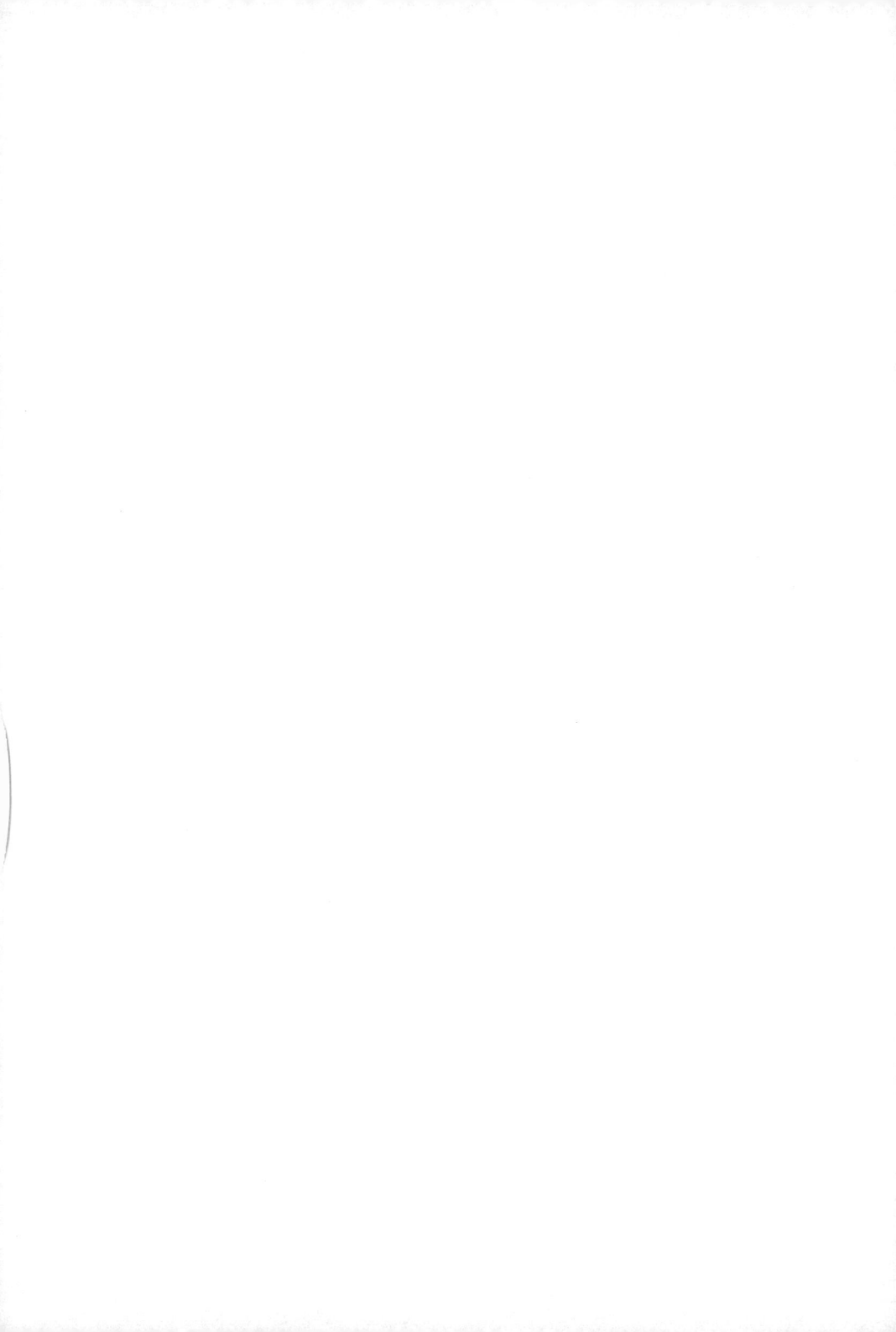

1

Systems Within Systems: Families in Society

> **Learning Objectives**
>
> - Recognise the importance of language in understanding mental health
> - Appraise the value of social constructionism
> - Identify the characteristics of family systems theory and ecological systems theory
> - Appreciate the usefulness of discursive approaches to analysis of family communication

Introduction

This chapter provides the foundation for the rest of the book by introducing the key theoretical and conceptual frameworks within which specific notions are presented and positioned. We also introduce the datasets that are drawn upon for the analysis in later chapters and give a brief explanation about the discursive analytic approaches that have been used to examine family communication within these settings. For transparency and reflexivity, we detail our own personal and professional positionality in relation to our interests and experiences of working in the field of family communication and mental health.

Language and Communication

There are different theories and ideas about language, and our intention here is to simply provide a basic introduction to the role of language as is important for working with families. Likewise, the literature and area of communication is a complex one and is multidisciplinary in contributions to knowledge, and we do not have space for that level of complexity. Our discussion here is intended only as an introduction to these broad concepts to lay a foundation for our book and the more practical focus it retains throughout the chapters.

We acknowledge that the arena of communication is a vast one, and communication is by no means restricted only to the words that pass between people. Within families, and within health services, the range of symbols, artefacts, and images that are part of how people communicate is sophisticated and nuanced. These symbolic representations are embedded in the ways that people communicate and the meanings that they apply and attribute, the shared understandings of symbols, rituals, and images, and the subtle ways in which representations are utilised with successive generations and across different cultures is a fascinating topic in its own right.

One area that many trainee practitioners will have been introduced to are the ways in which body language can affect the way that a message is received. For example, a practitioner may communicate with words that they are interested and attentive to a client's narrative, but contradict that message by inattentive body language, such as folded arms, reading notes, looking at the clock, gazing out of the window, looking at a computer screen or even texting whilst a client is speaking. All these actions are sending messages to the client; they are forms of communication. Clients themselves, in turn, may also communicate a clear message, not necessarily with words, but again, by their actions; they may come late, or miss sessions, or disengage completely. Less dramatically, teens and younger family members, in particular, may position themselves on the periphery of the conversation, may play with their phone, or fiddle with something in the room, they may have closed body language, and/or wear clothing that 'hides' them such as hats or hoodies covering their eyeline.

1 Systems Within Systems: Families in Society

Clothing itself is a vast area of symbolic communication. Less often talked about in training programmes, the clothing that we choose as practitioners is another powerful form of communication. Most people will be conscious that in a workplace setting, wearing formal or semi-formal clothing is appropriate, or a uniform for those uniformed professions. However, the general public are well trained through our media saturated global economy to be attentive to the cues or meanings that certain clothing and jewellery may communicate. A large watch or diamond ring, for example, definitely communicates wealth and status, as do certain recognisable brands and styles of designer clothing. For practitioners working with families who may be part of a different socio-economic group, it is worth asking ourselves the question, what are our clothes and accessories communicating? For the most part, building rapport with clients is aided by a sense of similarity, and points of connection may be deliberately sought as part of that therapeutic relationship-building stage. One way to potentially minimise a power differential between practitioners and family members is to be mindful of the kinds of messages that our clothing may communicate to those that we are working with.

We can marvel at the vastness of the ways our clothing, our behaviour, and the spaces in which we work can communicate messages to our clients before we even open our mouths. This is all important contextual information when working with families and practitioners need to be mindful of this aspect of communication. In this book, however, we restrict ourselves primarily to the area of language and semiotics, with which we are most familiar, and with which we have chosen to specialise, but nonetheless recognise the importance of all forms of communication and allude to that where appropriate. Within the world of discourse, there is a richness that becomes more and more fascinating and inspiring the more closely it is examined. It may not be as fascinating to others as it is to us, but we hope that to some extent at least you catch our passion for how the use of language in communication can do so many interactional activities. To that end, we use many extracts of transcripts taken from real-life interactions between mental health professionals and families to illustrate the discussion topics throughout this book.

One perspective on language is that it describes and mirrors reality and experiences. For example, in family situations, language may be used to describe thoughts, feelings, relations, activities, and behaviours. This perspective on language is that it is treated as a tool to communicate with others the reality of the world. Another perspective on language is that people use their words carefully and the way they describe and explain things are motivated by a desire to achieve a particular outcome. Whichever perspective we take, it is clear that language is performative, in that people engage in social actions such as complaining, complementing, disagreeing, inviting, assessing, and so forth. In family situations, language is used in all these ways between family members. As such, different perspectives on the same topic emerge as different people present their own versions. Therefore, instead of a singular reality, multiple perspectives can exist within the same space.

The position that we take in this book echoes this appreciation of the multiple facets and multiple perspectives that people engage with their reality from, and therefore hold what is referred to as a social constructionist epistemology.

> **Social Constructionism**
>
> Social constructionism is a perspective that advocates that human experience is not predetermined but is co-created between people as they use language, and meaning is historically, culturally, and socially mediated and agreed/or disagreed (O'Reilly & Kiyimba, 2015).

> **Epistemology**
>
> Epistemology refers to the theory of knowledge (Harding, 1987,) as well as the means of knowledge production (Soini & Kronqvist, 2011).

Epistemology relates to the ways in which knowledge becomes accepted as factual and publicly credible (Soini & Kronqvist, 2011). A social constructionist perspective on how knowledge is generated and perpetuated hinges on the way that people use language in their everyday interactions. For example, if a discourse of disharmony is dominant within a family, that form of language labels the types of interactions that family members have as typically fractured and in conflict. From a narrative therapy point of view, one of the tasks of the therapist would be to consider alternative narratives that would use different language to label and describe family dynamics. In this way, language can be used to create or recreate the kinds of reality that people experience.

Within society, social constructionism operates at different levels, and it is helpful for us to acknowledge both macro and micro social constructionism as they inform and influence each other. From a macro perspective, social constructionism relates to the power of language (Burr, 2003), to shape social structures (Gubrium & Holstein, 2008) and institutional practices (Burr, 2003). These social and institutional practices are embedded in cultural and historical narratives (Chen et al., 2011). From a micro perspective, social constructionism relates to the detail of everyday localised situated interactions (Gubrium & Holstein, 2008). In other words, how people in their daily conversations can reproduce macro societal discourses and iteratively perpetuate those dominant views. One of those discursive practices is the enactment of perspectives that stigmatise certain groups of people.

Stigma

Erving Goffman (1963) defined stigma as stereotyping the characteristics of certain groups of people in such a way that positions them as inferior. The consequences of being devalued through stigmatisation, according to Goffman, may result in rejection and isolation. Stigmatising attitudes and behaviours are influenced by the political, historical, and economic context (Corrigan & Miller, 2004). For those with mental health conditions who experience stigma and discrimination, this can significantly impact their quality of life and recovery pathway (Sartorius, 1998). Research has shown that stigma can increase symptoms associated with their condition (Hill & Startup, 2013) and can impact education or employment opportunities (Thornicroft et al., 2009) and may in some cases increase the risk of suicide (Thornicroft, 2011). There is growing evidence that sustained social discrimination is a factor in the shortening of telomeres which decrease life expectancy (Chae et al., 2014; Coimbra et al., 2020).

> **Telomere**
>
> Telomeres are protective caps at the end of DNA sequences. Chronic stress has been shown to speed up telomere shortening, which has been linked to acceleration of aging and aging-related diseases.
>   (Source: Chae et al., 2020)

Labelling

With the advent of the diagnostic manuals DSM and ICD came a structured way for medical professionals to categorise symptom clusters and assign a label to consistently identify appropriate treatment pathways to support families and individuals. Despite the honourable intentions and the utility of having standardised ways of diagnosing and treating mental health conditions, societal influences have reframed some diagnoses in a pejorative way. Thus, for those individuals who have been allocated a certain diagnostic label, they may experience social rejection due to the stigmatisation of mental ill health.

As a result, the sociologist Thomas Scheff (1966) developed his labelling theory, which provided an account for the ways in which social attitudes and reactions can influence accepted social norms. Scheff emphasised that stigma is a social construct with powerful social responses when people are labelled with certain conditions (Wallace, 2010). From this perspective, people within certain social contexts adopt the normative stereotyped ideas about mental health which are perpetuated through negative and discriminatory language (Weinstein, 1983). Notably, people are so influenced by social norms, they may also internalise the negative language themselves (e.g., O'Reilly et al., 2009; Rose et al., 2007). One of the things that practitioners working with families who experience stigma may be able to do is to challenge some of those internalised negative beliefs about mental health labels. By supporting family members to reject the pejorative social discourses and to embrace the benefits of having been assigned a diagnostic label, there is hope for those individuals to regain some control over how they present and experience themselves in social contexts.

One way to help families take control of how they are represented is to challenge the dominant individualistic notions of stigma and labelling. Instead of assigning potentially stigmatising labels to passive recipients, we are now better at recognising the social framework and political cultural context in which normality and deviance are positioned (Farrugia, 2009). Thus, although the early work of Goffman (1963) on stigma and of Scheff (1966) on labelling were particularly influential and, in some ways, advanced our thinking, we now have a wider understanding of the wider social and political influences on the social construction of pathology.

Pathology

Social constructionism is a way of understanding the social and psychological as established through social interpersonal processes (Georgaca, 2014). In relation to mental health, this has significant implications for how normality and pathology are positioned and understood (O'Reilly & Lester, 2017). From this viewpoint, therefore, there is a clear distinction between the biology of the disease and the social meaning of the condition or 'illness' (Eisenberg, 1977). This taps into arguments about universality where researchers and practitioners seek to understand whether mental health difficulties are experienced in the same way across cultures or different groups of people. The distinction in social construction between disease symptoms and their meaning is a useful differentiation, in the sense that it allows for certain elements of the experience to be acknowledged while also appreciating that the meaning of those experiences can be interpreted differently by different people. In family systems, taking this social constructionist position allows room for exploration of the experience and meaning making of the same situation by different family members.

In relation to mental health, one way to make sense of a family member's behaviour may be that their actions are 'symptoms' of a biological mental health condition. This has sometimes been referred to as the influence of 'nature' rather than 'nurture'. Another way of making sense of that behaviour, particularly in the case of children, is to understand it as the product of their environment, such as the behaviour of a child who has not been appropriately disciplined. These differences in meaning making from the same precipitating event illustrate how normality and pathology are socially constructed entities. There are various social and political forces that are influential from a macro perspective in determining which of these interpretations are preferred (Brown, 1995). A contentious area where this construction of normality and pathology occurs is in medical environments. For services engaging with families within the medical paradigm, language based on pathology and illness and deviance is common. However, services engaging with families from a sociological paradigm are more likely to mobilise language that draws on concepts of experience, meaning, perspective, and acceptable idiosyncratic differences. Thus, different professional training can mean that practitioners working with the same family are approaching the situation from different viewpoints and sometimes families do not fully understand the different roles and purpose of them. We propose that the social constructionist perspective that we offer is beneficial in reconciling these tensions.

> The social constructionism perspective helps us to understand that there is no single 'truth' and there may be contested versions of the same event by different family members.

As we move through the book, we acknowledge medical frameworks such as diagnostic criteria as being standard descriptive ways of communicating with other professionals who operate within the same paradigm and problematise this dominant discourse as being not the only way to conceptualise family difficulties. Even within the medical field, it is acknowledged that the existing constructs of mental health and illness are not fixed but are "heterogenous, changeable in shape that we can never establish fixed boundaries between them" (Frances, 2013, p. 16). In other words, establishing diagnostic categories of mental health conditions relies on communication between practitioners and agreement about the notion of mental health or illness. One of the aspects of medical language that we question is the negative and deficit-laden vocabulary (Walker, 2006) used to talk about people as broken or pathological, and thus medicine is invoked to 'fix' the person (O'Reilly & Lester, 2016). The social constructionism perspective that we provide throughout this book offers an alternative narrative to this pathologising discourse which allows for greater scope of framing the identity, experience, and meaning of the family interactions that we utilise in our exemplars. This is important as the pathologising language often associated with mental health conditions can configure roles for practitioners and their clients that may not be useful in most professions.

Social Meta-Narratives

Communication with families inevitably occurs within the situated context of a cultural, historical, economic, and political system. As such, even the smallest or most mundane conversations are influenced by these social meta-narratives. In making sense of mental health, there is therefore a need to account for the ways in which the interrelated educational, cultural, familial, social, and political systems intersect (Weare, 2000). While there are several theoretical perspectives, we introduce two influential theories to provide a helpful framework for making sense of communicating with families that are also foundational for the direction of the arguments presented through the book. First, we discuss Bronfenbrenner's (1979) ecological systems theory and second, we discuss Bowen's (1966) family systems theory.

Ecological Systems Theory

According to Bronfenbrenner's child development theory, there are five intersecting 'layers' of influence. These are (1) the immediate *micro-system* around the child which includes, family, school, peers, health service, and religious organisations; (2) the *meso-system* refers to the interactions between those elements of the micro-system, such as families communicating with schools; (3) the *exo-system*, consists of the wider influences such as the family's socio-economic status, the role of the media, and government policies; (4) the *macro-system* consists of ideologies and attitudes of the culture, including the wider social contexts, for example, living within a war environment; and (5) the *chrono-system* consists of the processes of change over time influencing the child, including changes on a micro or macro level, such as parental divorce, or wider social change. Importantly, when evaluating the cause and effect of one constitute component on another, the influence of these systems is not unidirectional, rather these systems dynamically influence one another.

In continuing the development of the theory, Bronfenbrenner (2005) advocated that children are to some extent active in their development and interact with the systems around them. In contemporary society, their development plays out in various ways and through different platforms. In a digital society, and one where children's rights are promoted in most countries (see United Nations, 1989), there are a multitude of modalities for children to develop and construct their identities and within the context of the five systems described. Thus, children are influenced by and simultaneously influence those systems and do not only sit as passive objects at the centre but play a partial active role.

Returning to our previous argument about the social construction and discourses of pathology, within that biomedical narrative, medical professionals often seek for the aetiology of a 'condition/disease', to ascertain appropriate 'interventions'. However, our argument is not only that pathology is a social construct perpetuated by dominant discourses but also that aetiology is non-linear because constructs of deviance and normality and their explanations are part of the wider multidirectional symbiotic ecosystem. Thus, communication with families in the context of mental health involves being mindful of this complex ecological system when considering issues of cause and effect or of blame and accountability.

Family Systems Theory

Bearing in mind all the wider influences on the family micro-system, it is incumbent to also recognise the unique interactions that occur within specific family groups. Each family has its own idiosyncratic ways in which the functioning of the family relies on reciprocal interdependence. Families often also develop dominant narratives about their family identity and about the constructed identities of various family members (Dallos, 1991). These narratives are perpetuated through patterns of conversational interactions that maintain relational circularity. For narrative therapists more specifically, these patterns can become a focus for positive deconstruction to allow the emergence of healthier or more adaptive ways of storying family dynamics.

As an emotional unit, the family profoundly impacts its members' actions and feelings as they seek to garner one another's approval, attention, and support and react to one another's needs, emotions, and expectations (Bowen, 1966; Dallos & Draper, 2010). Family systems theory focuses on the interactions between family members, as well as the ways in which those members relate to wider community, educational and healthcare systems (Watson, 2012). Watson noted that according to this perspective, the way an individual behaves is more to do with interpsychic rather than intrapsychic factors, such as hierarchies, boundaries, coalitions, loyalty conflicts, beliefs, projections, and systemic anxiety.

In recognising the value and influence of Bowen's family systems theory, we also acknowledge its genesis as intrinsically embedded within an individualistic Westernised perspective. As such, some of the values and ways of conceptualising family dynamics may not be as appropriate for different family constellations within collectivist cultures. With this caveat in mind, we introduce the core components of Bowen's theory as outlined by Winek (2010):

1. *Differentiation of self*: refers to the optimum level of individuation where there is an emotional connection with other family members without an unhealthy emotional fusion, enmeshment, or overidentification with others.
2. *An emotional triangle*: this represents the smallest stable network, whereby more than two people are required to alleviate anxiety within a family system.
3. *The family projection process*: this relates to the possibility of parents transmitting their anxiety or emotional concerns to the child and consequently seeking professional help for the child rather than addressing their own relationship difficulties.

4. *The multigenerational transmission process*: for Bowen, people seek out partners with a similar level of differentiation which over subsequent generations may lead to lower levels of differentiation and create the need for this pattern to be broken.
5. *An emotional cut-off*: emotional cut-off is an unhealthy way of managing family conflict which in the short term may manage anxiety and stress but ultimately lead to more problems.
6. *Sibling position*: the likelihood of youngest, middle, and elder children assuming certain roles within the family system due to differences in systemic factors, such as parental discipline, expectations, and so on.
7. *The societal emotional process*: the relationship between social and familial emotional processes whereby larger social issues like overpopulation and availability of natural resources bidirectionally influence the emotional stability of the family system.
8. *The nuclear family emotional process*: families can experience difficulties in four main areas which are emotional distance, problem behaviours in one of the members, impaired function of children, and intimate partner conflict.

When communicating with families within a Western framework, these eight components can be a helpful starting point in considering the complexity of the family system as a group of individuals who mutually influence and are influenced by one another. A system perspective considers that the family is more than the sum of its parts, noting that systems are self-organising, and members of a system produce their own pattern of behaviour over time for the purpose of nurturing and protecting its members (Watson, 2012). An important thing to bear in mind is that practitioners have evolved the conversation around systems thinking, and this is influential in modern practice with families (Dallos, 2006). For example, narrative approaches have located the way in which people pathologise within the family as not simply internal to that family system but drawn from a pool of culturally shared discourses (Dallos, 2004).

Throughout this book, in our analysis of conversations with families, we note that discourses are situated and contextual and that accounts are produced for certain purposes at certain times and therefore there is never one simple way of looking at a problem. Rather, individual members of families narrate problem discourses from their own perspectives which are influenced by these wider systemic factors. Family members may implicitly or explicitly draw upon wider socio-cultural narratives or external systems in their account-making practices.

The Construction of Reality Within Family Systems

The theoretical foundations of both systems theory and social constructionism are compatible, in the sense that they share several premises. Specifically, in both models, there is a focus on the way that meanings are mutually constructed within the dynamics of social interaction, and ideas are exchanged through joint actions (Dallos & Urry, 1999). Dallos and Urry argued that these two theories emphasise how individual experiences and characteristics are not static and ubiquitous across different contexts and settings but are fundamentally interpersonal and social. Family members use language to perform many 'speech acts', such as persuading, justifying, accusing, inviting, admiring, seducing, and so forth (Austin, 1962). As such, when talking about themselves or other family members, individuals construct their own and other people's identities through these rhetorical devices for certain purposes (Billig, 1987).

In the process of constructing the identities of another family member through language, people may engage in maintaining problem talk by reproducing dominant negative discourses about that person. The context of the family home is often the arena where certain kinds of discourses are perpetuated. Notably, both social constructionism and systemic theory make relevant the significance of contexts in relation to family interactions and dynamics (Dallos & Urry, 1999; Dallos & Draper, 2010). For example, family members may use different discursive repertoires in a home environment than in leisure, work, or school contexts.

Although none of the data in this book are based on practitioners using Narrative Therapy (NT) as an intervention, it is helpful to at least consider some of the foundational tenets of this approach, as it is also based on a social constructionist worldview. The core position of NT is that the problem is the problem. In other words, it is not the person that is the problem, but the person and the problem should be separated (White & Epston, 1990). From this philosophical position, the ways that people talk in families, and the words they choose, are understood as ways to "express self-reinforcing memories, thoughts, images, and feelings that form their perception of themselves and their world as narratives of life" (Ghavibazou et al., 2022, p. 2). Indeed, early experiences are viewed as being important, and Dallos (2006) contributed significantly to the field of narrative therapy through his explication of the relationship between early attachments and emotional experiences and how they influence the development and formation of family narratives. The stories or narratives that family members speak to one another become internalised, and form parts of mental rumination, or are re-used in conversations with others. The goal of narrative approaches to therapy is to support family members to explore alternative 'versions' of events or identities that have been constructed through these shared stories. This is usually done by considering additional aspects that may not have been mentioned, or may have been overlooked, and by modifying dominant discourses that may be skewed or biased, so that they become closer to reality (Payne, 2010).

Research Data

Throughout this book, we will refer to various research projects and the data generated from them to support the claims made, to demonstrate points, and as examples to illustrate meaning. Mostly these projects report on naturally occurring datasets. Naturally occurring activities happen in everyday life formally and informally. Similarly, naturally occurring texts are written materials that occur in everyday or institutional settings. When those activities are recorded or those texts are utilised for research purposes, they become referred to as naturally occurring data (Kiyimba et al., 2019). In other words, the naturally occurring activity happens regardless of whether a researcher harnesses it for analysis (Potter, 2002). The findings from these research projects have been identified through the inductive process of approaching data from the position of 'unmotivated looking' (Sacks, 1992).

> **Unmotivated Looking**
> Unmotivated looking refers to the general exploration of the data, engagement with those data without being encumbered with preconceived ideas or plans of what to look for, but instead to just see what is interesting or feels important.
> (Source: Sacks, 1992)

In addition, due to the applied focus of this book, we also include concepts and skills that would be familiar to practitioners in counselling, therapy, and helping professions, such as active listening, Socratic questions, and circular questions. In doing so, we at times take a deductive approach to illustrate examples of these skills using data from a range of sources.

About Our Projects

To help provide examples of our points, we draw on empirical data. Throughout our careers, we have been involved in many different research projects within the field of mental health. To help our readers to better engage with the materials in this book, we draw upon four of our research projects.

Family therapy projects: We undertook research into family therapy by recording naturally occurring therapeutic sessions. Our first family therapy project consisted of 22 h of family therapy video data with two practising family therapists (pseudonyms, Kim and Joe) and four families (pseudonyms, Clamp family, Niles family, Webber family, and Bremner family). Thus, the first family therapy project examples are represented in this book with these pseudonyms to anchor them as examples from that specific family therapy project.

Our second family therapy project consisted of recordings of therapy sessions with two families, where different members of the family were at times seen separately by the practitioner, and at times seen together. Thus, the second family therapy project examples are represented by the pseudonyms of the clinic that they were attending. These were named Oak

Clinic and Beech Clinic, and where we use data examples from this data corpus, we identify the project using those pseudonyms.

Mental health assessment project: We undertook research into the practice of mental health assessments in a UK Child and Adolescent Mental Health Service (CAMHS). This involved video recording 28 different families. The practising professionals consisted of psychiatrists, psychologists, occupational therapists, psychotherapists, and community psychiatric nurses. Each assessment was approximately 90 min long. Where we use examples from this specific project, we refer to the family identifier number that they were given for the project (i.e., family one, family two, etc.).

Suicide prevention project (LOSST LIFFE): We interviewed a range of practitioners from various occupational groups, including charity helpline call takers, mental health professionals, police officers, and police staff, teachers, educational psychologists, academics, faith leaders, from the UK, New Zealand, and Guyana. The focus of the interviews was on their work with self-harm and suicide, their challenges in the work, and their views and perspectives. This project is only pertinent to our chapter on risk and data examples are labelled appropriately to indicate this.

All the projects had appropriate ethical approval and governance. All parties, families, children, professionals, and other parties provided informed consent (or assent). We use pseudonyms throughout to protect the identities of those participating.

Analytic Approaches

The research projects we utilise in this book are all qualitative and are in keeping with our social constructionist position and predominantly use the language-based approaches to analysis. These include:

- Conversation analysis, an analysis of the sequential unfolding of talk in particular settings to examine the ways in which certain utterances are influenced by prior turns of talk and shape subsequent responses (Sacks, 1992).
- Discourse analysis is the study of talk and text as mechanisms for the implementation of social actions such as blaming, complaining, justifying, inviting, and so forth (Potter, 1996).

- Discursive psychology, the application of discourse analysis to psychological concepts to explore the constructed nature of psychological processes, such as memory, attitudes, and perception (Edwards & Potter, 1992).

The common feature of each of these discursive approaches to analysing data is an awareness of the performative function of language. In other words, when people say things, they simultaneously engage in a social action, such as complementing, blaming, or complaining. When we analyse extracts of conversation between practitioners and family members, one of the key areas of interest is to explore how people treat other people's talk as performing an interactional function. The data extracts are presented in a transcription format called the 'Jefferson' approach which allows the analyst to consider *how* things are said as well as *what* has been said (Jefferson, 2004). Due to the focus on language, the standard transcription convention used throughout this book is quite detailed and includes representation of how things are said, such as speed, increased volume, and emphasis (Jefferson, 2004). An outline of these representational symbols and their meanings can be found in appendix A at the end of the book and are taken from seminal texts on the approach. Throughout the book, then we will be using many examples of data from our research projects. This transcription convention is typical for researchers using conversation and discourse analysis. We introduce you to this style in the following section, to give an idea about the nature of the analysis throughout the book and to illustrate how the theories we introduced map against real world data.

Introductory Examples of Discursive Analysis of Family Systems

The following data extract is presented as an example of how a family in family therapy use discursive repertoires that are appropriate to a formal institutional context. Simultaneously, in serving the purposes of justifying, accounting, and explaining, family members narrate incidences of conversations that have occurred previously in other contexts, including at home with other professionals and in their child's school. Therefore, their discursive practices reflect both attention to the 'in here' current family therapy interaction and draw on 'out there' examples of other interactions to support and verify their claims. In relation to family systems theory, this is a common practice as family members typically discuss matters related to their internal interactional dynamics as well as interactional dynamics with external agencies such as educational and healthcare providers and the wider community (Watson, 2012). We provide a good example of how dispositional attributions are constructed within the 'in here' interaction of family therapy (taken from Parker & O'Reilly, 2012, p. 464).

Niles family

```
Father:   <we've got t' sort> (.) o:r get some medication or
          somet t' calm 'is temper ↓down (.) cuz 'e's ↑schizo
```

In this extract, the father refers to his son as 'schizo' (characterising him as schizophrenic) and in doing so locates the child's behaviour as being internal and dispositional. This is further consolidated by his request to '*get some medication or somet to calm his temper down*', which additionally positions the child as 'mentally ill' and in need of psychiatric medication. In social constructionist terms, this is an example of how another person's behaviour is constructed in a particular way using discursive rhetorical devices for a specific purpose. Although the father is ostensibly projecting a dispositional account onto his son, his doing so occurs in a family therapy session where his son is present in the room, and it could therefore potentially be considered inappropriate to be talking about his son in those terms in front of him. The following extract exemplifies drawing on 'out there' systems and contexts to perform a social action (taken from O'Reilly & Parker, 2014, p. 304).

Clamp family

```
Father:      I think it might ['ave been 'cause the police =
Mother:                       [and last night
Father:      = arrested me 'at the house and everythin' they do
             it <at the wrong time> when the kids are there and
             that ↓lot
Therapist:   I think >for all of you< it's been a very difficult
             time and e::r
```

In this extract, the parents' complaint in the current interaction is about the behaviour of the police in a prior interaction that occurred outside the therapy room: in the family's social world. The trajectory of the current therapy conversation has in part focused on what is or is not appropriate to talk about in front of the children. At this point, the father moves the focus of conversation away from what is happening 'in here' to report an incident of inappropriateness of what had happened 'out there'. There are four elements to the complaint: first is informational, that is a description of what is inappropriate, that is, being arrested, second is locational, identifying the place where the incident took place, that is, at the house, third is temporal, that is the time the incident occurred, that is, at the wrong time, and fourth is the personal, the person who performed the act, that is, the police (see O'Reilly & Parker, 2014). By describing an external event, the father constructs the presence of the children during the event as objectionable rather than the arrest itself. Strangely in projecting blame onto an external third party, the social action the father performs is to protect his own identity as a good parent. Throughout this book, we use the discourse analysis term 'social action'. What we mean by this is that when people say things, they perform actions at the same time, such as blaming, excusing, and complimenting. Each of these actions that are accomplished through the words people speak are called social actions.

Throughout this book, we encourage you to engage with a series of reflective activities to help you understand, process, and translate some of the content in relation to your own practice. We recommend that you keep a reflective diary as you read through the book and use this as a space to address the reflective activities and make notes. We invite you to undertake the activity in Box 1.1.

> **Box 1.1 Activity on Language**
>
> **Reflective activity**
> **Language and families**
> An important thing to think about in discourse analysis is that people do not just say things because they are 'facts' or because what they are saying is 'true'. People tend to say things to create an impression in someone else's mind.
> Think about how individuals use language to construct their own and other people's character and how they attach meaning to different events or incidents. What kinds of things do people say about other family members that create an impression of that family member having a particular character trait? What impression might they be trying to create by doing that?

Author Positionality

Any text is imbued with the positionality of its author, the theoretical frameworks that underpin their work, and a reflexive appreciation of how personal and professional experiences shape the writing. Here, we provide the reader with some information about our history and how we came to write this book.

Michelle: I first became interested in the field of mental health during my childhood mostly because of my autistic brother. It was a difficult time during those early years where my parents recognised that he required support but had a 'battle' to acquire the diagnosis. Diagnosis led to family engagement with various mental health professionals and charities. There were certainly frustrating times during this period where my family had difficult conversations, especially with social services and education providers trying to meet his complex needs, as well as emotional periods where his behaviour would be challenging. Thus, as a teenager I volunteered with various mental health charities as I wanted to better understand autism, but also some of the co-occurring mental health conditions he experienced. It was this personal association living with someone diagnosed with autism, as well as being engaged with professionals with expertise that encouraged and motivated me to learn more and pursue my own career in that direction. During those volunteer placements, I learned a great deal from different professionals I encountered and came to appreciate the importance of family and family-based interventions. I started to recognise how my own family dynamic functioned and the importance of working together to support my brother's needs. It was these experiences that motivated my career in psychology, beginning with a BSc with honours psychology degree, followed by a master's degree, and then a PhD. During those study years, I continued the voluntary work and took on placements with clinical psychologists, educational psychologists, art therapists, and special educational needs schools. These practical opportunities for dialogue with experienced professionals provided me with foundational understanding of the application of psychology in practice. It was also during this study time that I began my research career, and I was exposed to a range of methodological approaches. During my master's degree, I came to learn discourse analysis and conversation analysis, which was consolidated during my PhD. The training in discursive methods provided a way of understanding family interactions and mental health conversations that laid the foundation and motivation for my career in applied research and qualitative methods. This led to my status as a chartered psychologist in health and associate professor of communication in mental health, working for both the University of Leicester and Leicestershire Partnership NHS Trust.

Nikki: My family, like most people, was the formative environment that had a huge influence on shaping who I am now, my interests, and the career path I have chosen. From a very young age, I recall words, language, and communication being central. Our living room was lined with books, and my mother's voracious appetite for reading was easily absorbed by my inquisitive mind. She was a speech and language therapist, and on days when I was off sick from school, I would occasionally go with her to the clinics where she worked. I quickly learned that her job, that she loved so much, was not just about helping children pronounce words clearly, but about helping family members of all ages understand and communicate with one another. A small thing to many, such as being able to communicate a desire for a cup of tea, could be a great breakthrough for one client, and the joy everyone experienced in making that possible was evident. My father was a larger than life, good humoured, sociable man, and he had a knack of being able to make himself understood to people from all ages and backgrounds, whether they spoke English or not. With a series of nods, smiles, and enthusiastic hand gestures, he would always quickly make friends and be able to build a rapport with others everywhere he went. So, communication was everywhere, and even in our small family, I learned about how we as humans are social creatures. When I came to study social psychology at university, I first learned about speech as an action and was fascinated to explore further how people use words to do all manner of things. My undergraduate psychology dissertation was a reflection on the ethical dilemmas inherent in utilising rhetorical discourse strategies in religious preaching. Drawing on the then new discipline of discursive psychology for my PhD, I was curious about the ways that adults, young people, and children communicate differently and how that played out in family interactions. My longstanding appreciation of words, language, and communication dovetailed neatly with my newfound academic knowledge about discourse analysis and psychology. Even now as a clinical psychologist, the ability to use words to help people share their inner words, to show care and validation, and to help them heal still fascinates and motivates me.

The partnership: Our connection began at Loughborough University where we were both PhD students within social sciences. At the time, there was a vibrant community of academics who were working within the field of discursive approaches to data analysis, and we were part of the Discourse and Rhetoric Group (DARG). The characteristics of the Loughborough School were a combination of discourse and rhetoric, discursive psychology, feminist discourses, and conversation analysis. This foundation has informed and influenced much of the development of our work since then. Following graduation, there were several years where we followed different career trajectories with Michelle focusing on an academic path and Nikki taking a clinical route. An encounter by chance a few years later in a car park of a CAMH service led to reconnecting and beginning working collaboratively. Initially, we met regularly in person to write together until Nikki moved to another part of the UK and we continued our partnership by virtual meetings. More recently, Nikki emigrated to Aotearoa, New Zealand, but despite time zone differences and distance, we have continued to work together. Our research on family interactions and our pedagogical roles in training clinical practitioners help us to ensure that our work is firmly grounded in practice. The quality of our outputs thus benefits from not only our long-standing friendship but also our complementary skill sets that enable us to combine a strong academic foundation, with clinical application.

Final Thoughts

Working with families requires attention to the power of language and meanings within social interactions. For some practitioners, it may be new to consider how powerful specific ways of talking and asking questions can be in terms of how families respond. We hope from reading this chapter the value of using naturally occurring data and discursive approaches to analysing those data are apparent. By being reflexive about our own positionality and transparent about our theoretical allegiances, we seek to model a way of approaching our practice and encourage the reader to consider their own positionality as they work through the book. To support this process, we include several suggestions for reflective practice in each chapter.

We summarise the key messages from the chapter in Box 1.2.

Box 1.2   Key Points

- Language is a vehicle to perform social actions.
- Through language, normality and pathology are constructed.
- Social constructionism is an established theoretical framework to understand how both different perspectives and positions are created and maintained.
- Family systems theory recognises the influence of different systems on a child, recognising the interactions within the family and wider social systems.
- Ecological systems theory positions the nuclear family within wider social cultural systems and the interactions between those.
- Throughout this book, we draw upon several research projects as examples to illustrate our points.
- Due to the complexity of social and cultural influences on families, awareness of one's own reflexive positionality is invited.

References

Austin, J. (1962). *How to do things with words*. Oxford University Press.

Billig, M. (1987). *Arguing and thinking: A rhetorical approach to social psychology*. Cambridge University Press.

Bowen, M. (1966). The use of family theory in clinical practice. *Comprehensive Psychiatry, 7*, 345–374.

Bronfenbrenner, U. (1979). *The ecology of human development: Experiments in nature and design*. Harvard University Press.

Bronfenbrenner, U. (2005). The bioecological theory of human development. In U. Bronfenbrenner (Ed.), *Making human beings human: Bioecological perspectives on human development* (pp. 3–15). Sage.

Brown, P. (1995). Naming and framing: The social construction of diagnosis and illness. *Journal of Health and Social Behavior, extra issue*, 34–52.

Burr, V. (2003). *Social constructionism* (2nd ed.). Routledge.

Chae, D., Nuru-Jeter, A., Adler, N., Brody, G., Lin, J., Blackburn, E., & Epel, E. (2014). Discrimination, racial bias, and telomere length in African American men. *American Journal of Preventive Medicine, 46*(2), 103–111.

Chae, D., Wang, Y., Martz, C., Slopen, N., Yip, T., Adler, N., et al. (2020). Racial discrimination and telomere shortening among African Americans: The coronary artery risk development in young adults (CARDIA) study. *Health Psychology, 39*(3), 209.

Chen, Y., Shek, D., & Bu, F. (2011). Applications of interpretive and constructionist research methods in adolescent research: Philosophy, principles, and examples. *International Journal of Adolescent Medicine and Health, 23*(3), 129–139.

Coimbra, B., Carvalho, C. M., Ota, V., Vieira-Fonseca, T., Bugiga, A., Mello, A., et al. (2020). A systematic review on the effects of social discrimination on telomere length. *Psychoneuroendocrinology, 120,* 104766.

Corrigan, P., & Miller, F. (2004). Shame, blame, and contamination: A review of the impact of mental illness stigma on family members. *Journal of Mental Health, 13*(6), 537–548.

Dallos, R. (1991). *Family belief systems, therapy and change: A constructional approach.* Open University Press.

Dallos, R. (2004). Attachment narrative therapy: Integrating ideas from narrative and attachment theory in systemic family therapy with eating disorders. *Journal of Family Therapy, 26*(1), 40–65.

Dallos, R. (2006). *Attachment narrative therapy.* McGraw-Hill Education.

Dallos, R., & Draper, R. (2010). *An introduction to family therapy: Systemic theory and practice* (3rd ed.). Open University Press.

Dallos, R., & Urry, A. (1999). Abandoning our parents and grandparents: Does social construction mean the end of systemic family therapy? *Journal of Family Therapy, 21,* 161–186.

Edwards, D., & Potter, J. (1992). *Discursive psychology.* Sage.

Eisenberg, L. (1977). Disease and illness: Distinctions between professional and popular ideas of sickness. *Culture, Medicine, and Psychiatry, 1,* 9–23.

Farrugia, D. (2009). Exploring stigma: Medical knowledge and the stigmatisation of parents of children with autism and developmental delay. *Autism, 13,* 375–387.

Frances, A. (2013). *Saving normal: An insider's revolt against out-of-control psychiatric diagnosis, DSM-5, big pharma, and the medicalisation of ordinary life.* Harper Collins.

Ghavibazou, E., Hosseinian, S., Abdollahi, A., & Ghamari Kivi, H. (2022). Effectiveness of narrative therapy on adult attachment styles and expressivity in women experiencing low marital satisfaction. *Counselling and Psychotherapy Research, 22*(4), 853–860.

Georgaca, E. (2014). Discourse analytic research on mental distress: A critical overview. *Journal of Mental Health, 23*(2), 55–61.

Goffman, E. (1963). *Stigma: Notes on the management of a spoiled identity.* Prentice Hall.

Gubrium, J., & Holstein, J. (2008). The constructionist mosaic. In J. Holstein & J. Gubrium (Eds.), *Handbook of constructionist research* (pp. 3–12). Guilford.

Harding, S. (1987). Introduction: Is there a feminist method? In S. Harding (Ed.), *Feminism and methodology: Social science issues* (pp. 1–14). Indiana University Press.

Hill, K., & Startup, M. (2013). The relationship between internalized stigma, negative symptoms and social functioning in schizophrenia: The mediating role of self-efficacy. *Psychiatry Research, 206*(2–3), 151–157.

Jefferson, G. (2004). Glossary of transcript symbols with an introduction. In G. Lerner (Ed.), *Conversation analysis: Studies from the first generation* (pp. 13–31). John Benjamins.

Kiyimba, N., Lester, J., & O'Reilly, M. (2019). *Using naturally occurring data in health research: A practical guide*. Springer.

O'Reilly, M., & Kiyimba, N. (2015). *Advanced qualitative research: A guide to contemporary theoretical debates*. Sage.

O'Reilly, M., & Lester, J. N. (2017). *Examining mental health through social constructionism: The language of mental health*. Palgrave.

O'Reilly, M., & Lester, J. N. (2016). Introduction: The social construction of normality and pathology. In M. O'Reilly & J. N. Lester (Eds.), *Handbook of adult mental health disorders* (pp. 1–19). Palgrave Macmillan.

O'Reilly, M., & Parker, N. (2014). 'She needs a smack in the gob': Negotiating what is appropriate talk in front of children in family therapy. *Journal of Family Therapy, 36*(3), 287–307.

O'Reilly, M., Taylor, H., & Vostanis, P. (2009). "Nuts, schiz, psycho": An exploration of young homeless people's perceptions and dilemmas of defining mental health. *Social Science and Medicine, 68*, 1737–1744.

Parker, N., & O'Reilly, M. (2012). 'Gossiping' as a social action in family therapy: The pseudo-absence and pseudo-presence of children. *Discourse Studies, 14*(4), 1–19.

Payne, M. (2010). *Couple counselling: A practical guide*. Sage Publications.

Potter, J. (2002). Two kinds of natural. *Discourse Studies., 4*(4), 539–542.

Potter, J. (1996). *Representing reality: Discourse, rhetoric, and social construction*. Sage.

Rose, D., Thornicroft, G., Pinfold, V., & Kassam, A. (2007). 250 labels used to stigmatise people with mental illness. *BMC Health Services Research, 7*, 97–104.

Sacks, H. (1992). In G. Jefferson (Ed.), *Lectures on conversation* (Vol. I & II). Basil Blackwell.

Sartorius, N. (1998). Stigma: What can psychiatrists do about it? *Lancet, 352*, 1058–1059.

Scheff, T. (1966). *Being mentally ill: A sociological theory*. Aldine de Gruyter.

Soini, H., & Kronqvist, E. (2011). Epistemology—a tool or a stance? In H. Soini, E. Kronqvist, & G. Hüber (Eds.), *Epistemologies for qualitative research* (pp. 5–8). Centre for Qualitative Psychology.

Thornicroft, G. (2011). Physical health disparities and mental illness: The scandal of premature mortality. *British Journal of Psychiatry, 199*(6), 441–442.

Thornicroft, G., Brohan, E., Rose, D., Satorius, N., & Leese, M. (2009). Global pattern of experienced and anticipated discrimination against people with schizophrenia: A cross-sectional survey. *Lancet, 373*, 408–415.

United Nations. (1989). *Conventions on the rights of the child*. UN.

Wallace, J. (2010). Mental health and stigma in the medical profession. *Health, 16*(1), 3–18.

Walker, M. (2006). The social construction of mental illness and its implication for the recovery model. *International Journal of Psychosocial Rehabilitation, 10*(1), 71–87.

Watson, W. (2012). Family systems theory. In *Encyclopedia of human behavior* (2nd ed., pp. 184–193). https://www.sciencedirect.com/topics/medicine-and-dentistry/family-systems-theory

Weare, K. (2000). *Promoting mental, emotional and social health: A whole school approach*. Routledge.

Weinstein, R. (1983). Labeling theory and the attitudes of mental patients: A review. *Journal of Health and Social Behaviour, 24*(1), 70–84.

White, M., & Epston, D. (1990). *Narrative means to therapeutic ends*. W.W. Norton.

Winek, J. (2010). *Systemic family therapy: From theory to practice*. Sage.

2

Family Dynamics and Constructs

> **Learning Objectives**
> - Recognise the intricacies of family constitution
> - Allow space for families to be self-determining about roles and identities
> - Critically assess the concepts of resilience and vulnerability
> - Demonstrate awareness of the different ways that practitioners can work effectively with family systems

Introduction

The goal of this chapter is to introduce the broad socio-cultural framework within which family constellations are positioned. We invite a critical inquiring stance of the reader that reflexively interrogates the world view prevailing within the professional context in which they work. In guiding the reader through this chapter, we encourage attention to the ways in which families self-define their roles and relationships; thus, promoting a family-centred stance. In developing this chapter, it is not our intention to explore in detail any specific modalities of working with families and neither is this a scholarly academic thesis on the socio-political development of the family system throughout history. Rather, in this chapter, we have simply introduced some of the core arguments and contributions from the evidence as a heuristic to provide a foundation for the practical chapters that follow.

What Constitutes the Family?

In seeking to define what constitutes a family, a dominant discourse has been to consider 'family' in relation to its structural properties. From this perspective, there are a wide range of different structural types that make up different kinds of family groupings depending on culture, context, history, and situation. There may be biological, economic, legal, or social ways of identifying familial structures in terms of identifying who belongs to a family group or household, and sometimes these are conflated. Even within the structural way of thinking about families, it is important to recognise that structures can change. Indeed, as more diverse forms of families are emerging in our society, it becomes ever more necessary to build an understanding of how family dynamics influence the ways in which children and young people can engage with mental health services to support them (Anakwe et al., 2020).

An alternative discourse is to consider family in terms of function. A good example of this is to consider 'parenting' as a role or function within the family system, rather than trying to define too categorically who the parents are. The people who function in the parenting role may be different over a period as the family structure trajectory evolves. Family member identities may need to be reconfigured and renegotiated over time as individuals form initial and subsequent intimate partner relationships and children from those relationships navigate transitions into new 'hybrid' or 'blended' family groupings. It is not unusual in modern family systems for children to co-habit with siblings who have different biological parents who are co-parented by several adults, some of whom will co-habit in the same household, with others physically located elsewhere (Sanner et al., 2020). These complex co-parenting systems are also subject to change over time as adults dissolve and form new relationships. In other words, it is important to treat and understand families as dynamic rather than static structures and therefore as capable of assuming shifting and transitional trajectories over time (Johnston et al., 2020).

> Kinship care is an example of various extended family members functioning as parents for those children (United Nations, 2010), and is often the preferred option for children who cannot reside with biological parents (Australian Institute of Health and Welfare, 2021; McCartan Bunting, Bywaters et al., 2018; Wu and Snyder, 2019).

The Social Construction of the Family

The very notion of the 'family' is not straightforward to define, and there are arguably multiple meanings of the concept. Furthermore, family is defined at different levels, by the individuals within the unit, the community, institutions, society, and political structures. Across these domains, the way that families are defined has been shaped by history and culture. In this way, the family is not a fixed or defined concept but a dynamic one that is socially constructed. Thus, all the different levels may define family in slightly different ways. For example, there may be an institution or political structure that defines family in a specific way, but the individuals within the 'family' may include certain people within what they see as their unit but exclude others from it. The composition of what they determine as family may be different from legal or official constructions of it. However, the legal frameworks will be an influence on practice, and thus it is important to be mindful of any legal constraints such as the requirement to have consent from both parents to work with the child when parents are separated.

> It is important (within legal constraints) to listen to family members and respect their own construction of what family means to them.

Terminology or language used, such as 'aunt', 'uncle', 'cousin', and 'brother/sister', is part of their family constellation of discourses that may be attributed to people who may or may not be biologically connected to the individual. The use of family discourse to refer to non-biological members is one way that people can demonstrate a familial type of relationship with that person. As a practitioner, it will be important to ascertain some information about the construction of the family from the members' perspective in terms of:

- Who is who?
- What roles do they play?
- What do they mean to the child?
- What support does that person offer the child?
- Are there any possible risk factors associated with that person?

To illustrate some of the ways in which families narrate their own familial identities and relationships, we provide some examples of data where family members are describing some of these dynamics. A fundamental aspect of parenting is making decisions about the children's well-being and engaging in discipline to set boundaries. In the following extract (from previously unpublished data), the stepfather (referred to as 'Dad') describes the difficulties of having an equal right with the children's mother to implement these aspects of parenting.

Webber family

```
Dad:    It's more (0.6) I mean like when it comes down to like
        (0.2) decisions with the kids (0.2) it it's hard for
        like for me and Mandy to agree because like like I'm
        sayin' Mandy's the mother to all of them
FT:     Hum
Dad:    Where I'm not biologically th[e father =
FT:                                  [Sure (.) sure
Dad:    = to all of them so you know what I mean [I can't =
Mum:                                             [Just
        biological to Stuart aren't you
Dad:    = I've got a split (0.6) thing so I could easily turn
        round and say well look you know solve Daniel's problem
        give him a bloody good hiding =
```

The 'Dad' in this family system is only biologically connected to one of the children (Stuart) and the other three children, including Daniel whose problematic behaviour is being discussed in this setting, are his children by marriage *'I'm not biologically the father to all of them'*. In this professional setting of family therapy, the practitioner is working with the parents to find a solution to Daniel's behaviour. However, the stepfather constructs his role in addressing the problem as peripheral, positioning the mother as being the one who ought to—and more appropriately—take more responsibility; *'you know solve Daniel's problem, give him a bloody good hiding'*. There are several possible ways to understand the stepfather's identity management of his role:

- The possibility that he may feel that he does not have the right to discipline his stepson but would like to.
- He may be abdicating responsibility for discipline because it is so challenging.
- He may be navigating a position where he is mitigating blame by distancing himself.

For the practitioner working with a family like this, an understanding of the ways in which family groupings describe their own internal relationship dynamics is an important starting point. This provides a foundation for exploration of some of these identity management possibilities and the ways in which they might be challenged or worked with to facilitate more harmonious family relations.

From a child's perspective in a situation where there is a biological parent who is no longer co-habiting with the family group, there may be different relational dynamics to work with. In the following example, the child describes his frustration and hurt resulting from his efforts to contact his non-resident biological father to no avail (taken from Kiyimba & O'Reilly, 2018, p. 151).

Family 18 (Prac = Psychiatrist)

```
Prac    So you said he was a prick
Child   Yeah
Prac    how did you (.) ↓come to that conclusion or how did you:
```

```
Child    because (.) I've (0.34) always ↑tried to like get in
         touch with 'im and (0.66) make a (.) relationship but
         he's always just like (0.31) never (0.30) tried or
         bother t' (1.71) meet me ↓or: (.) talk
```

In this example, the child described his biological father using the derogatory term of 'a prick'. In seeking to understand the child's use of this terminology, the psychiatrist asks, *'how did you come to that conclusion'*. The child describes taking the initiative to contact and build a relationship with his father, without success as the father did not reciprocate. In this case, the core challenge for the practitioner appears to be one of attachment and the management of the sense of abandonment that the child seems to be experiencing. As a practitioner, it is clearly not possible to change the circumstances or a non-present father, and thus the focus can only be on the child and his feelings. Understanding the child's perspective and his expectations of what family 'should' be is helpful regarding supporting the child's psychological adjustment to the situation.

Sociology of the Child

The concept of what a family has undergone changes across history and culture and in a similar way so has the notion of the child and childhood. Despite historical and cultural variation, there is generally universal agreement that childhood is a developmental phase of maturation and learning where there is a need for guidance and protection. The length of time that 'childhood' is acknowledged may vary across cultures, as is the transition from childhood to adulthood and the various ceremonies and rites of passage that may mark that transition. Additionally, expectations vary from culture to culture about what a child is expected to do. From a historical point of view, the introduction of mandatory education was only formalised in the late 1800s, at which point children were gathered together in classroom settings (Karim, 2015). These environments where children were gathered together provided a different environment from the family where children could engage with their peers. Additionally, this provided a mechanism for observation that led ideas about normative development by having the opportunity for comparison of children of a similar age with one another (Karim, 2015). From a Western perspective, children were historically viewed as lacking competency or agency, however, more modern views of childhood acknowledge children as capable of contributing to decisions that may affect them (James & Prout, 2015).

The Victorian notion of the child being 'seen but not heard' has now been replaced by an emphasis on child-centred practice. A child-centred approach requires practitioners to view the child's needs as central to the institutional task, recognising that regardless of chronological age, the child has a right to a voice (O'Reilly et al., 2021). Children are recognised as having rights, especially regarding their physical and mental health (see United Nations, 1989) and children are now considered to be active agents who can and should have influence over decisions about aspects of their lives (Montreuil & Carnevale, 2016). We invite the reader to complete the reflective activity in Box 2.1 which may highlight differences between your own experiences of childhood and your current professional context.

> **Box 2.1 Reflective Activity on Childhood**
>
> **Reflective activity**
>
> **Reflecting on childhood and practice**
>   Here, we invite you to address the following three activities and write down your answers as part of your reflective journal and, where possible, discuss your responses with colleagues.
>
> 1. Reflect on your own experience of childhood.
> 2. Reflect on the current dominant social narratives about childhood.
> 3. Consider your own professional context and how your own experiences of childhood and current dominant narratives influence the way that you practice.

Vulnerability and Resilience Factors in the Family

Resilience has often been argued to be a quantifiable measurement, either intrinsic to an individual or behaviourally learned (Agaibi & Wilson, 2005). It can refer to a person's ability to 'bounce back' or return to their usual level of functioning after a stressful period (Richardson, 2002). Vulnerability factors are those that might impede a person's ability to return to that usual level of functioning. Within the literature, the primary focus tends to be on defining factors that make an individual more resilient or vulnerable. However, in the context of developing mental health conditions, a good way of thinking about resilience and vulnerability is that on a spectrum they are two elements that require balance. Thus, in the context of working with family systems, it can be helpful to think about the family group as somewhere on the spectrum of resilience and vulnerability.

Definition	
Resilience: The ability to 'bounce back' and cope with challenging life circumstances	Vulnerability: Personal, familial, social, and structural factors that impede the ability to cope with challenging life circumstances

Disruption and Resilience

Transitions occur in multiple forms throughout the lifespan. For children, transitions, such as the birth of a sibling, move to a new school or neighbourhood, illness or death of grandparents, or older siblings leaving the home, occur in addition to structural and functional reconfigurations as parents may separate and form new relationships. The immediate micro-system around the child (Bronfenbrenner, 1979) is disrupted or perturbed during these transitions. Any disruption to the family micro-system creates a challenge for all involved and children especially may need additional support to navigate and cope with the cognitive and emotional disruptions these changes cause (Hovmand et al., 2022).

While changes to family structures are not new, the complexity of family life including multiple stepfamilies adds further layers of challenges that need to be considered (Brown et al., 2015). It may be helpful not to think of the family trajectory as purely linear but to consider these changes as dynamic, reciprocal, and cyclical, whereby the family system is in a constant state of flux and needing to find ways to achieve an equilibrium (Hovmand et al., 2022; Richardson, 2011). In other words, a new equilibrium needs some organisation, as families re-organise (their roles, ways of relating, understandings) to achieve that equilibrium, and the old family patterns and practices require new ones for the new organisation.

To find a state of equilibrium, it is typically the small everyday interactions that can be the most powerful. Indeed "even relatively simple interactions between an individual child, their family, and the school as their social environment can generate complex dynamics" (Hovmand et al., 2022, pp. 145–146). Hovmand et al. argue then, that the adults fulfilling the function of parenting provide key modelling examples to the children of how to manage adaptation and distress in a familial feedback loop. Where adults are themselves caught in negative or dysfunctional patterns or strategies for managing difficulties, children may need additional supports to develop more adaptive and positive responses.

As we noted in opening this section, one of the arguments that have been proposed is that children need to develop resilience to cope with adversity and need to be supported in this development. Resilience has been constructed as the capacity to withstand and rebound from life challenges (Walsh, 2016a, 2016b) and "recover quickly from difficulties" (Oxford English Dictionary, 2018, n.p.). Much of the literature has characterised resilience as either intrinsic to the person or behaviourally learned (Agaibi & Wilson, 2005). However, it may be better understood as a combination of intrinsic qualities and cognitive and behavioural strategies that can be learned (Kiyimba, 2020) and is arguably influenced by early attachment (Phillips & Dallos, 2006). Thus, resilience can be described as an adaptive consequence of positive human development (Caffo & Belaise, 2003), involving a dynamic process of learned and innate strategies to cope in the context of adversity (Masten & Cicchetti, 2016). Notably, most explorations of the concept of resilience have been framed within an individualistic perspective, but more recent thinking on the matter has highlighted the significance of family and wider systems (e.g., Theron, 2016; Ungar, 2011). That is, resilience processes are viewed as occurring within mutual networks, and social and cultural structures (Theron, 2016), and are considered more in terms of social ecologies of resilience moving responsibility away from individuals to the wider environment (Ungar, 2011).

As we have shown, then, often the notion of resilience refers to the child's ability to be resilient and cope with adversity in their life. However, more contemporary understandings of resilience recognise that resilience is not simply dispositional to the child but rather reflects the resilience of the systems around the child and acknowledges how structural inequalities, multiple disadvantages, and societal influences will contribute to resilience. This is important in noting that individualistic ideas can oversimplify the complexity of adversity (Ungar, 2005). In other words, it is valuable to consider contextual factors relating to how individuals engage with their environments, as part of a young person's developmental pathway (Ungar & Liebenberg, 2011). This supports the argument that resilience is better conceptualised as a process that is intrinsically tied to the young person's relationships, attachments (Chiang et al., 2018), and cultural influences (Theron et al., 2015).

Of relevance for practitioners working with families is the notion of family resilience, which is a systemic perspective on the family as a functional unit (Walsh, 2003). Systems theory proposes that life challenges impact the whole family and depending on the ways in which key members of the family respond, cumulative stressors can negatively impact family functioning (Walsh, 2016a). Family resilience has been defined as the capacity of the family to rebound from stressful life challenges in ways that draw upon the family's resourcefulness (Walsh, 2016b). For children, the wider family, including extended family and friends, can provide emotional and practical support (Rose et al., 2022), which are key aspects of the family resilience model (Walsh, 2016b).

Vulnerability Factors

Similarly, the related concept of vulnerability has typically been positioned in the literature as a static and intrinsic quality of an individual or a group. Arguably, though, a more helpful way of understanding vulnerability is to think of it as dynamic and contextual rather than dispositional (Nordentoft & Kappel, 2011). A key concern for practitioners working with families is to be attentive to the possibility of risk or harm for family members. A way of describing this might be to use the language of vulnerability to understand a person's current situation as posing a more imminent potential for harm. Shivayogi (2013) uses the concepts of 'capacity to protect oneself' and to 'make informed choices' as characteristics typically lacking in vulnerable people. If we apply these concepts in a more dynamic fashion, there may be times and contexts where a family member is less able to protect themselves or make informed choices.

An assessment framework that is often used within the helping professions and particularly useful for collecting information about vulnerability and risk factors is the 4 P's model (Weerasekera, 1996). Often a fifth 'P' is added in professional practice, which is the 'presenting problem'. In the following table, therefore, we provide the original four P's as outlined by Weerasekera (1996), but we also add the fifth P, of presenting problem for the sake of completion, and these are outlined in Table 2.1.

When considering the first P in this table, which is the presenting problem, this can be an area that different family members have a different perspective on. Alternatively, the family may have a dominant narrative that is maintained and re-presented in informal family conversations. This dominant narrative may become part of the 'performance' of the problem in the contexts of professional help-seeking.

The second P in the table (predisposing factors) is often understood with reference to biological and hereditary factors within the family, such as a propensity towards heart disease or mental health difficulties. The opposite of this is the perpetuating factors which are typically environmental (although not always), such as living in poverty, unhelpful peer-relationships, poor nutrition, i.e., factors that contribute to the maintenance of the difficulties. Historically, biological, and environmental factors have been considered in a binary way however new evidence demonstrates that biological markers are environmentally influenced. For example, the field of epigenetics shows us that DNA is not as deterministic as previously thought but can be influenced by the environment, including the mother's diet during pregnancy and stress (Kiyimba, 2016; Painter et al., 2008). Evidence also shows that the way in which DNA is

Table 2.1 The five P's

	Description and examples		
The five P's	Biological	Psychological	Social
Presenting	Somatic presentations such as headaches and stomach aches may be part of the presenting problem	Examples such as anxiety or depression are typical presentations for people seeking help from mental health services	Behavioural factors are often the most tangible and noticeable aspects of the presenting difficulty
Predisposing	Genetic factors that might make someone more vulnerable to physical or mental health conditions	Dysfunctional cognitive, behavioural, and emotional responses learned within the family environment	Socio-economic context of the family that may disadvantage members
Precipitating	Current or recent health problems within the family	Current or recent factors causing anxiety or stress	Current or recent social and/or relational challenges such as conflicts with others
Perpetuating	On-going chronic physical or mental health challenges	On-going chronic ways of thinking and reacting to circumstances that are maintaining unhelpful cycles	On-going chronic social difficulties such as conflicts or poor relationships
Protective	Constitutional good health	Helpful coping strategies for maintaining cognitive and emotional balance	Supportive family and/or peer relationships

read can be altered with supportive social interactions, nutrition, physical activity, and relaxation techniques (Behm, 2012).

Overall, the second, third, and fourth P's in this assessment framework speak to ascertaining potential vulnerability factors, whereas gathering information about the fifth P is important in understanding what intrinsic and extrinsic factors may support individual and family resilience. Arguably, the resilience factors of the fifth P have not attracted as much attention as the vulnerability factors captured in the second, third, and fourth P. However, Richardson (2002) noted that a shift towards strengths-based practice which highlights a greater focus on protective or resilience factors in assessment.

> Supporting the whole family, can in turn help and support the individual members.

Following an assessment using the five P's, a model that may be quite useful for practitioners working in the field of mental health, is the stress vulnerability model (see Zubin & Spring, 1977). According to this model, the greater the number and intensity of challenging events, the greater the likelihood is of someone being vulnerable to becoming unwell. We represent this in Fig. 2.1 taken from Kiyimba (2020, p. 198).

According to Lazarus (1993), a person's ability to cope is a balance between the internal and external demands and the person's perceived resources to meet those demands. Together with Folkman, Lazarus created the transactional model of stress, proposing that people become unwell when the demands outweigh their resources (Lazarus & Folkman, 1987). This is represented in Fig. 2.2 (taken from Kiyimba, 2020, p. 174).

To maintain a balance between demands and resources, Duerden (2018) proposes two potential types of intervention:

1. *Problem-focused change:* to reduce the problem. To alleviate or remove the internal or external challenge.
2. *Resource-focused change:* to increase the coping resources. To support or develop greater strategies to manage the challenges.

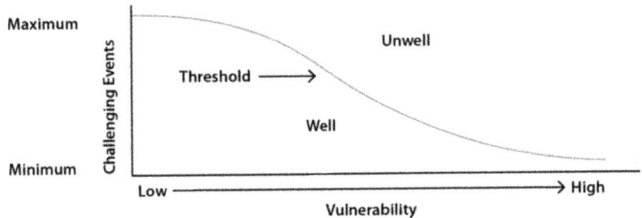

Fig. 2.1 Stress vulnerability model

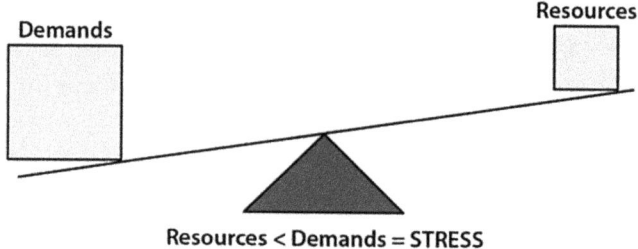

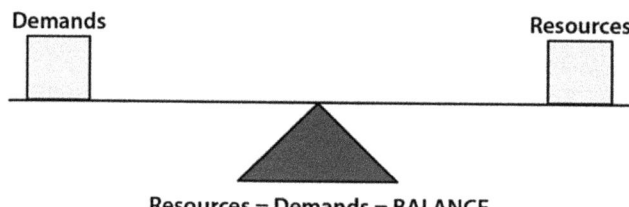

Fig. 2.2 Transactional model of stress

You may be in a position in your practice where you can facilitate or help the family with *problem-focused change* or it may be the case that your role enables you to help the family with *resource-focused change*. We encourage you to think about this further as you engage with the reflective activity in Box 2.2.

> **Box 2.2 Reflective Activity on the Transactional Model of Stress**
> Reflective activity
>   Reflecting on the transactional model of stress in practice
>   Here, we invite you to think about whether you can facilitate problem (demand) or resource-focused change in your professional role.
>
> 1. To what extent are you able to alleviate or lessen the demands on the family?
> 2. To what extent are you able to strengthen or increase the resources of the family?
> 3. What challenges might there be if family members do not know how to access or use their resources?

For children, adverse historical events are likely to increase vulnerability to mental health difficulties. However, historical events cannot be changed, and the challenge for family mental health practitioners is to consider what resources can be put in place to enable children's coping and resilience in the wake of what has happened in the past. The term 'adverse childhood events/experiences' (ACEs) is commonly used to describe several highly stressful or traumatic experiences that children may encounter. These are described in Table 2.2.

There are numerous studies that demonstrate that the larger the number the ACEs that the child experiences before their 18th birthday, the greater the risk of negative consequences in the child's development (Kiyimba, 2020). Indeed, research illustrates that childhood abuse, neglect, and family dysfunction typically occur together (Rosenberg et al., 2007). For practitioners, therefore, it is important to recognise how different kinds of adversity in childhood are "deeply intertwined"

Table 2.2 Overview of ACEs

ACE	Description
Physical abuse	Parent or known adult causing physical harm or injury to the child
Sexual abuse	Another individual older than the child inappropriately touching in a sexual way or intercourse
Emotional abuse	Insulting, humiliating, or making derogatory comments by an adult towards the child
Physical neglect	Not providing sufficient food and nutrition, clean clothes, or access to healthcare
Emotional neglect	Circumstances whereby the child feels unloved, unsupported, and unimportant
Mental illness	Whereby a member of the family has severe depression, mental illness, or engaged in a suicide attempt
Parental absence/loss	A parent is lost through divorce, abandonment, death, or other reason
Substance abuse	Parent or caregiver engages in problem uses of alcohol or drugs
Violence against the mother/stepmother	The frequent witnessing by the child of physical violence against their mother from another person
Having a relative incarcerated	Where the child has someone in the household sent to prison

(Merrick et al., 2017, p. 19). Unhelpful or maladaptive coping strategies, such as drinking or smoking, or taking drugs, may be used by adolescents and young adults as a strategy for stress reduction (Dembo et al., 1992). A key role for practitioners working with families where children (and potentially their parents) have experienced ACEs is to support them in establishing emotional regulation strategies that are helpful and resilience-building.

Given the more recent context of the global pandemic of COVID-19, it is worth noting that the additional restrictions imposed during the lockdown periods added additional pressures and strains to families (Cluver et al., 2020). The parenting challenges of home schooling and social distancing were also compounded by juggling work from home for some, economic pressures for most, and for some there were also redundancies (Gallagher & Wetherell, 2020). Some researchers argue that the profound impact on everyday family life caused by the complex responses to COVID-19 created considerably more stress within families, which in turn may have actually exacerbated or added to children's adverse experiences such as abuse, neglect, and interpersonal violence (Fegert et al., 2020; Mahase, 2020).

Working with Families in Mental Health

There are many ways in which families may be involved or included in work with a person within the family who has mental health difficulties. Broadly speaking, the ways in which families might be involved fall roughly into four domains:

1. To communicate with the family to acquire more information about how the individual family member with the mental health difficulty is in other contexts and settings and/or what coping or management strategies they are currently using.

2. To engage with family members around decisions about interventions for the family member with the mental health difficulties. This includes discussions about medication, inpatient admission, behavioural activities at home, nutrition, and exercise.
3. Sometimes families may need support practically or financially, such as respite care or families may benefit from psychoeducation about a particular mental health difficulty of their loved one.
4. The fourth aspect may be that members of the family are directly involved in a psychological intervention or treatment process. This kind of direct involvement is referred to as family-based psychological interventions (FBPI) (Carr, 2020).

In the literature, sometimes family members supporting someone with a mental health difficulty are referred to as carers. Importantly for the best outcomes for family members with mental health difficulties, a collaborative process between healthcare professionals, family members and the individual being treated is established. This dynamic interaction is sometimes referred to as the 'triangle of care' (Worthington et al., 2013). One corner of the triangle is the client, the second is the family, and the third is the professional helper. Notably, the aspect of the triangle where the professional helper sits may be constituted of several different practitioners from different professional sectors who may have either overlapping or competing agendas. These multiple influences may need to be navigated. In addition, the family corner of the triangle is also likely to be made up of various individuals, again with different perspectives.

However, family-based psychological interventions are based on the principle that family members are a valuable therapeutic resource and can include couple therapy, family therapy, and parent-assisted therapy focusing on children (Wampler et al., 2020). Studies consistently indicate that these FBPIs are more effective in addressing relationship problems than individual therapy (Carr, 2019, 2020; Riedinger et al., 2017). Specifically, FBPIs have been shown to be effective for working on attachment problems, child maltreatment, child and adolescent behaviour disorders, and eating disorders (Carr, 2020).

> The way in which family-based psychological interventions work is by helping family develop more functional and supportive relationships and better problem-solving strategies (Carr, 2022).

Final Thoughts

This chapter has introduced key concepts pertinent to the book in terms of what constitutes a family. Using extracts of data from family interventions, we have discussed the complexity of the ways in which families identify and dispute family roles and relationships. The importance of keeping this in mind as a practitioner is to allow families to be self-determining about what constitutes their family constellation and who is part of that. This can be helpful when conducting assessments to ascertain vulnerability and resilience factors within the family system. We have briefly discussed the use of the four/five P's model as a helpful assessment framework and have highlighted the impact of adverse childhood events (ACEs) on child mental health outcomes. For practitioners working with children in families, an awareness of the cumulative impact of ACEs can inform thoughtful and well-informed interventions that account for such risk factors. The value of working with families in a collaborative way to support individual members' mental health outcomes is expanded further in the practitioner box, Box 2.3. by Clement Chihota.

Reflecting on the key themes that have been discussed in this chapter, we are reminded of the intricacies of family dynamics and how internal and external factors symbiotically impinge on family wellbeing. For practitioners working with families, there is a great need to be sensitive to the intersectionality between the professional agenda of the institution, the needs of the family system, and the individual family member who is being supported. Often this family member is a child or young person,

Box 2.3 Practitioner Voice, Clement Chihota

Practitioner voices
Clement Chihota
Lecturer

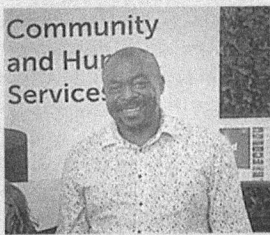

Clement Chihota (currently a lecturer in Social Work, Community, and Human Services at Federation University Australia) shares his experiences of working with children, young people and their families in the Child Youth and Family Services (Now Oranga Tamariki).

In my previous role as a Child Protection Social Worker in the Child Youth and Family Services (now Oranga Tamariki), I learnt that there was no set template for defining the family unit. In fact, I had to set aside my own preconceptions of what the family is—or should be like—and work with the families available to my clients. Thus, for the twin babies who were born to a single, teenage, immigrant mother, 'family' was that teenager plus a 30-something-old grandmom who was hardly available because she struggled with mental health issues. This was their family—and the family that I needed to work with! I also learnt that every family had its own 'home-grown' map of reality—and a trajectory, strong like a current, that carried the children along. I discovered ways of 'flowing along' with such currents, while also actively creating alternative channels that might lead to more positive outcomes. A clear 'no-no' in my work were attempts to flow against these family currents. Such attempts were futile as they not only instigated resistance but also often proved disorienting (if not alien) to the children/young people one was trying to help. In summary, I learnt that (a) every family is unique—and there is no universal template that qualifies what can (or cannot) be defined as a family unit; (b) every family unit has its own unique construction of 'reality'—and a trajectory that is shaped by this visualisation of reality. The practitioner needs to understand and work within this current, and only then can they find alternative channels that may lead to better futures for their clients.

(continued)

> **Box 2.3 (continued)**
>
> I left the Child Youth and Family Services just when the Tuituia assessment framework was being rolled out. Presented as a triangle, the Tuituia framework prioritised the voice and experiences of the child (or young person). It also explored parenting capacity and investigated ways of increasing this capacity to promote the safety and wellbeing of the child. Finally, the framework also explored material, social, and emotional resources that could be harnessed to advance the safety and wellbeing of the child and their family.
>
> My greatest 'take away', after working for almost three years in the Child Youth and Family Services, was that my role was not just to work with families. Rather, it was to work within the structures and dynamics of each individual family unit.

> **Box 2.4 Key Points**
>
> - What constitutes a family is socially, historically, culturally, linguistically, and dynamically constructed.
> - An alternative perspective to the binary conceptualisation of resilience and vulnerability was proposed as a spectrum.
> - The biological and environmental predisposing and perpetuating factors for family wellbeing were discussed using the model of four P's.
> - The importance of assessing adverse childhood events was highlighted in relation to increased vulnerability to mental health difficulties for those with a greater number.
> - The triangle of care and the value of collaborative relationships between health practitioners, family members/carers, and the individuals being supported were discussed within the context of different approaches to family work.

and it is helpful to bear in mind that the child is not an island. In other words, the child is raised within multi-systemic partnerships and influences, and the roles of different systems are important when working with a family. We summarise the key messages from the chapter in Box 2.4.

References

Agaibi, C., & Wilson, J. (2005). Trauma, PTSD, and resilience: A review of the literature. *Trauma, Violence and Abuse, 6*(3), 195–216.

Anakwe, A., Majee, W., Keller, K., & Jooste, K. (2020). Family structure diversity: Views from rural community leaders and implications for youth engagement. *Community Development, 51*(2), 157–171.

Behm, J. (2012). Rogers revisited: The genetic impact of the counseling relationship. *Ideas and Research You Can Use, 1*(1), 1–8.

Bronfenbrenner, U. (1979). *The ecology of human development: Experiments in nature and design*. Harvard University Press.

Brown, S., Manning, W., & Stykes, J. (2015). Family structure and child wellbeing: Integrating family complexity. *Journal of Marriage and Family, 77*(1), 177–190.

Caffo, E., & Belaise, C. (2003). Psychological aspects of traumatic injury in children and adolescents. *Child and Adolescent Psychiatric Clinics of North America, 12*(3), 493–535.

Carr, A. (2019). Family therapy and systemic interventions for child-focused problems: The current evidence base. *Journal of Family Therapy, 41*, 153–213.

Carr, A. (2020). Evidence for the efficacy and effectiveness of systemic family therapy. In K.S. Wampler, R.B. Miller, & R.B. Seedall (Eds.), *The handbook of systemic family therapy* (pp. 119–146, vol. 1). Wiley.

Chiang, J., Chen, E., & Miller, G. (2018). Midlife self-reported social support as a buffer against premature mortality risks associated with child abuse. *Nature Human Behaviour, 2*, 261–268.

Cluver, L., Lachman, J. M., Sherr, L., Wessels, I., Krug, E., Rakotomalala, S., Blight, S., Hillis, S., Bachman, G., Green, O., Butchart, A., Tomlinson, M., Ward, C. L., Doubt, J., & McDonald, K. (2020). Parenting in a time of COVID-19. *Lancet, 395*, 10231. https://doi.org/10.1016/s0140-6736(20)30736-4

Dembo, R., Williams, L., Wothke, W., Schmeidler, J., & Brown, C. (1992). The role of family factors, physical abuse, and sexual victimization experiences in high-risk youths' alcohol and other drug use and delinquency: A longitudinal model. *Violence and Victims, 7*(3), 245–266.

Duerden, T. (2018). Mindfulness: Potentially traumatising or detraumatising. In *'Minding the gaps' gaps' conference*. Retrieved from http://integratedmindfulness.com/mindingthegap2017/

Fegert, J. M., Vitiello, B., Plener, P. L., & Clemens, V. (2020). Challenges and burden of the coronavirus 2019 (COVID-19) pandemic for child and adolescent mental health: A narrative review to highlight clinical and research needs in the acute phase and the long return to normality. *Child and Adolescent Psychiatry and Mental Health, 14*(1), 1–11.

Gallagher, S., & Wetherell, M. (2020). Risk of depression in family caregivers: Unintended consequence of COVID-19. *medRxiv*. https://doi.org/10.1101/2020.06.15.20131532

Hovmand, P., Calzada, E., Gulbas, L., Kim, S., Chung, S., Kuhlberg, J., et al. (2022). System dynamics of cognitive vulnerabilities and family support among Latina children and adolescents. *Clinical Child and Family Psychology Review, 25*(1), 131–149.

James, A., & Prout, A. (2015). Introduction. In A. James & A. Prout (Eds.), *Constructing and reconstructing childhood: Contemporary issues in the sociological study of childhood* (classic ed., pp. 1–5). Routledge.

Johnston, C., Cavanagh, S., & Crosnoe, R. (2020). Family structure patterns from childhood through adolescence and the timing of cohabitation among diverse groups of young adult women and men. *Developmental Psychology, 56*(1), 165–179.

Karim, K. (2015). The value of conversation analysis: A child psychiatrist's perspective. In M O'Reilly and J.N. Lester (Eds.), The Palgrave handbook of child mental health: Discourse and conversation studies (pp. 25–41). Palgrave Macmillan.

Kiyimba, N. (2020). *Trauma-informed mindfulness: A Practitioner's guide for one-to-one work*. University of Chester.

Kiyimba, N. (2016). *Developmental trauma and the role of epigenetics* (pp. 18–21). BACP Healthcare Counselling and Psychotherapy Journal.

Kiyimba, N., & O'Reilly, M. (2018). Reflecting on what 'you said' as a way of reintroducing difficult topics in child mental health assessments. *Child and Adolescent Mental Health, 23*(3), 148–154.

Lazarus, R. (1993). Coping theory and research: Past, present, and future. Fifty years of the research and theory of RS Lazarus: An analysis of historical and perennial issues. *Psychosomatic Medicine, 55*, 234–247.

Lazarus, R., & Folkman, S. (1987). Transactional theory and research on emotions and coping. *European Journal of Personality, 1*, 141–169.

Mahase, E. (2020). Covid-19: EU states report 60% rise in emergency calls about domestic violence. *British Medical Journal, 369*, m1872. https://doi.org/10.1136/bmj.m1872

Masten, A., & Cicchetti, D. (2016). Resilience in development: Progress and transformation. In D. Cicchetti (Ed.), *Developmental psychopathology* (Vol. IV, 3rd ed., pp. 271–333). Wiley.

Merrick, M., Ports, K., Ford, D., Afifi, T., Gershoff, E., & Grogan-Kaylor, A. (2017). Unpacking the impact of adverse childhood experiences on adult mental health. *Child Abuse & Neglect, 69*, 10–19.

Montreuil, M., & Carnevale, F. (2016). A concept analysis of children's agency within the health literature. *Journal of Child Health Care, 20*(4), 503–511.

Nordentoft, H., & Kappel, N. (2011). Vulnerable participants in health research: Methodological and ethical challenges. *Journal of Social Work Practice, 25*(3), 365–376.

O'Reilly, M., Dogra, N., Levine, D., and Donoso, V. (2021). Digital media and child and adolescent mental health: A practical guide to understanding the evidence. .

Oxford English Dictionary (2018). Oxford English dictionary online version. https://en.oxforddictionaries.com/definition/resilience.

Painter, R., Osmond, C., Gluckman, P., Hanson, M., Phillips, D., & Roseboom, T. (2008). Transgenerational effects of prenatal exposure to the Dutch famine on neonatal adiposity and health in later life. *British Journal of Obstetrics and Gyneacology, 115*, 1243–1249.

Phillips, S., & Dallos, R. (2006). Attachment and adolescent depression: The impact of early attachment experiences. *Attachment & Human Development, 7*(4), 409–424.

Richardson, G. (2002). The metatheory of resilience and resiliency. *Journal of Clinical Psychology, 58*(3), 307–321.

Richardson, G. (2011). Reflections on the foundations of system dynamics. *System Dynamics Review, 27*(3), 219–243.

Riedinger, V., Pinquart, M., & Teubert, D. (2017). Effects of systemic therapy on mental health of children and adolescents: A meta-analysis. *Journal of Clinical Child and Adolescent Psychology, 46*, 880–894.

Rose, L., Taylor, E., Di Folco, S., Dupin, M., Mithen, H., & Wen, Z. (2022). Family dynamics in kinship care. *Child & Family Social Work, 27*, 635–645.

Rosenberg, S., Lu, W., Mueser, K., Jankowski, M., & Cournos, F. (2007). Correlates of adverse childhood events among adults with schizophrenia spectrum disorders. *Psychiatric Services, 58*(2), 245–253.

Sanner, C., Ganong, L., & Coleman, M. (2020). Shared children in stepfamilies: Experiences living in a hybrid family structure. *Journal of Marriage and Family, 82*(2), 605–621.

Shivayogi, P. (2013). Vulnerable populations and methods for their safeguard. *Perspectives Clinical Research, 4*(1), 53–57.

Theron, L. (2016). Toward a culturally and contextually sensitive understanding of resilience: Privileging the voices of black, south African young people. *Journal of Adolescent Research, 31*, 635–670.

Theron, L., Liebenberg, L., & Ungar, M. (Eds.). (2015). *Youth resilience and culture*. Springer.

Ungar, M. (2011). The social ecology of resilience: Addressing contextual and cultural ambiguity of a nascent construct. *American Journal of Orthopsychiatry, 81*, 1–17.

Ungar, M. (Ed.). (2005). *Handbook for working with children and youth: Pathways to resilience across cultures and contexts*. Sage Publications.

Ungar, M., & Liebenberg, L. (2011). Assessing resilience across cultures using mixed methods: Construction of the child and youth resilience measure. *Journal of Mixed Methods Research, 5*(2), 126–149.

United Nations. (1989). *Conventions on the rights of the child*. UN.

Walsh, F. (2003). Family resilience: A framework for clinical practice. *Family Process, 42*, 1–18.

Walsh, F. (2016a). *Strengthening family resilience* (3rd ed.). Guilford Press.

Walsh, F. (2016b). Family resilience: A developmental systems framework. *European Journal of Developmental Psychology, 13*(3), 313–324.

Wampler, K., Miller, R., Seedall, R., McWey, L., Blow, A., Rastogi, M., & Singh, R. (Eds.). (2020). *The handbook of systemic family therapy, 4 vols*. Wiley-Blackwell.

Weerasekera, P. (1996). *Multi-perspective case formulation: A step towards treatment integration*. Krieger Publishing Company.

Worthington, A., Rooney, P., & Hannan, R. (2013). *The triangle of care-carers included: A guide to best practice in mental health care in England* (2nd ed.). The Carers Trust.

Zubin, J., & Spring, B. (1977). Vulnerability: A new view of schizophrenia. *Journal of Abnormal Psychology, 86*(2), 103–126.

3

Forming and Maintaining Good Relationships

> **Learning Objectives**
>
> - Recognise the value of strong therapeutic relationships
> - Critically assess the benefits and challenges of alignment
> - Identify circumstances in which rupture might occur
> - Reflect on the ways in which social and contextual conventions impinge on turn-taking practices and the conversational experience of interruptions
> - Consider how different members might be treated in the institutional interaction

Introduction

When conversing with families, there are several variables to negotiate to successfully maintain beneficial alignment in relationships with each family member. The aim of this chapter is to explore some of the challenges to the endeavour of establishing therapeutic relationships. The evidence base critically questions the extent to which the relationship between the practitioner and family members is potentially more beneficial, or at least significantly important, than the intervention type specifically. As such the importance of therapeutic rapport, whether face-to-face or on a virtual platform, is necessary to take time to consider. Different cultures have different perspectives on how much attention is given to the relationship versus the task components of professional engagement with families. However, we argue that the relationship is the vehicle for the task to be achieved, and therefore there is great value in giving attention to and prioritising the relationship factors in working with families.

The Therapeutic Relationship

Although there is a huge amount of information about different communication strategies and techniques that are beneficial in mental health professional relationships, the overriding evidence suggests that the relationship itself has more influence of the successful outcome than the specific interventions (Kiyimba, 2020a). Early reviews of the literature demonstrated that 30% of positive change is due to therapist attributes such as warmth, congruence, and empathy, with the "main curative component is the nature of the therapeutic relationship" (Lambert & Barley, 2001, p. 357). Notably, this parallels the three core conditions of person-centred care which are empathy, congruence, and unconditional positive regard (Rogers, 1957). A more recent review of 16 meta-analyses conducted by the American Psychological Association (APA) Task Force on Evidence-Based Relationships and Responsiveness (specifically related to psychotherapy) concluded that the value of several relationship factors is related to positive therapeutic outcomes, and we outline several of these in Table 3.1 (DeAngelis, 2019).

Establishing and Maintaining Alignment

The conversational device that different parties use to position themselves in relation to their interlocutor's message is called alignment (Atkinson et al., 2007; Nofsinger, 1991). The notion of alignment in relation to

Table 3.1 DeAngelis (2019) findings from 16 meta-analyses on therapeutic relationships

Relationship factor	Description
Fostering mutuality and collaboration	It is argued that there needs to be mutuality in the therapeutic relationship to promote equality in the partnership
Agreeing therapeutic goals	It is important that there is partnership in developing the therapeutic goals and agreement on what they might be and how to achieve them
Being flexible and responsive	Therapists require skills to tailor treatments to individuals and consider the cultural background, therapy preferences, spiritual beliefs, gender identity, and so forth and need to be responsive to that individual
Using feedback	A technique for facilitating the therapeutic relationship is to gather feedback from the client and incorporate that into the treatment process
Repairing rupture	There are different factors that can disrupt therapy alliance, but it is important to resolve these ruptures to achieve better outcomes
Handling negative emotions	It can be challenging for therapists to repeatedly address negative states and not become frustrated
Promoting effective endings	At the end of therapy, there are different techniques to close the therapeutic relationship, including mutual discussions, facilitating future coping strategies, reflecting on therapeutic gains, and expressing pride in the progress made

family conversations is like the idea of establishing rapport (Spencer-Oatey, 2004), where rapport is experienced as a sense of solidarity or connection (Spencer-Oatey & Žegerac, 2017). The value of alignment activity is that it is a way to display mutual understanding in situ (Tecedor, 2016). According to Ohta, there are two main ways of building relationship alignment which are acknowledgements and assessments (Ohta, 2001). Ohta described acknowledgements as being the interlocutor indicating receipt of the message and being ready to continue, whereas assessments were described as requiring an expression of personal position. Notably, in multi-party family interactions, it is necessary for the practitioner to respect and value individual members and to build and maintain alignment with everyone, so that each person has a sense of belonging and involvement (Anderson, 2001).

To examine the interactional process of alignment in more detail, we focus on three examples. The first is the role of active listening in maintaining the therapeutic relationship.

> **Active Listening**
> The process of displaying clearly to the speaker that what has been said has been heard and can include skills such as summarising and reflecting.

The second examines how the colloquial activity of gossiping might function in a professional context as an alignment-building strategy between a family member and practitioner.

> **Gossiping**
> Gossiping is defined as being triadic whereby a non-present third party is talked about (Michelson et al., 2010), typically in a negative way (Noon & Delbridge, 1993).

The third considers how extreme forms of assessment (extreme case formulations: Pomerantz, 1986), can be used to build alignment in situations where there are apparent age or cultural differences that need to be navigated.

> **Extreme Case Formulation**
> Extreme cases are when people utilise terms that emphasise an extreme version, either the maximum or minimum of something (e.g., always, never, definitely, everybody, and nobody). They strengthen a claim or propose the validity of one (Pomerantz, 1986).

Language and Active Listening

To maintain the therapeutic relationship, the language used by the practitioner has importance. Notably, different professions working with families are trained in different ways, and yet being reflective about practice is a mainstay for many. Arguably, reflecting on language use can be a helpful mechanism for thinking about the therapeutic relationship and managing difficult conversations with family members. A skill that many counsellors and therapists learn as a core component of their training is active listening.

Active listening is when an interlocutor demonstrates involvement in the interaction by verbally indicating an understanding of the speaker's message (Tecedor, 2016). The key components of active listening involve reflecting and summarising (Geldard & Geldard, 1998). Geldard and Geldard defined reflecting as identifying core content details of what the speaker has said and reporting those words back to them for confirmation. They defined summarising as pulling together the thread of key points in what the speaker has said to demonstrate understanding. At this point, it becomes relevant for the hearer to offer either agreement or disagreement with the formulation offered, which is demonstrated in the following data example.

Child (J) and Counsellor (C)—taken from Hutchby (2005, p. 18)

```
J:  It's really hard because my dad tells me t'do one thing
    and my mum tells me tuh do the other=.hh=an' it feels a
    bit like I showed you last week, .hh with my da:d saying
    do this and wi' mum saying do this an' I don't know
    what t' do:.
    (0.7)
C:  So y- y- you get told t'do two different things [at ] the=
J:                                                   [Yeh]
C:  =same ti:me.
```

This example is typical, in that usually it is the family member that gives a longer more detailed explanation of a family interaction, and the practitioner offers a summarised or shorter reflective overview. In this case, the counsellor summarises what the child has said, in a simple phrase 'you get told two different things' to which the child agrees in overlap 'yeh'.

In making choices about which are the salient points to reflect or summarise to the hearer, there are various options (Hutchby, 2005). Using conversation analysis to look at transcripts of these kinds of conversations, it is possible to identify the results of making one choice of phraseology over another (Peräkylä, 1995). The practical accomplishment of active listening is a demonstration of how the practitioner has formulated the client's narrative in a way that is relevant to the professional interactional context (Hutchby, 2005). When working with families, it is common for family members to describe numerous situations or instances to the practitioner, and the skill of active listening is one by the practitioner that can synthesise this material into a brief professionally relevant summary that is endorsed by the family members. When done well, providing a summary or reflection of what someone has said can build the therapeutic relationship and rapport, because the speaker feels heard and understood. This is also referred to as the development and maintenance of therapeutic alignment.

Alignment Through Professional 'Gossiping'

We have titled this section 'professional gossiping' in respect of a paper we wrote published by the same name (Parker & O'Reilly, 2012). The key features of everyday gossiping are that the action is triadic (Michelson et al., 2010), evaluative (DiFonzo & Bordia, 2007), and usually negative (Noon & Delbridge, 1993). Gossip is triadic in everyday conversation in the sense that there is a speaker, a hearer, and a person being talked about who is not present (Foster, 2004). By speaking evaluatively and negatively about a non-present third party, gossiping serves the function of building an alignment between the speaker and hearer. In a similar way, in a professional context, a speaker and hearer may build alignment by talking in a (usually) negative way (i.e., 'gossiping') about a third party. In our family therapy data, the 'talked about' third party was present and part of the social interaction. We note that while discussing a third party builds alignment between two members of the interaction, it potentially excludes the overhearing third party. Therefore, interactional effort needs to be made to (re)include the overhearing third party to ensure alignment with one member of the family does not exclude alignment with another member of the family. The following data extract demonstrates one way in which this occurs.

Example Clamp family (taken from Parker & O'Reilly, 2012, p. 468)

```
FT:     What's it li↓ke hearin' yer mum an' dad (.) and me
        talkin' about things that you do?
        (5.5)
FT:     Does that bother you?
Phil:   ((Shakes head))
FT:     No?
```

Here, we can see the therapist orienting to the preceding minutes of conversation whereby the mother and father were providing him with information about their son Philip's behaviour with a negative overtone and negative examples. In giving space to the parents to express their perspective, the therapist builds a therapeutic alignment with them. However, the risk is that this potentially causes a disalignment between the therapist and the child. To correct and rebalance the alignment structure within the multi-party discourse, the therapist works to bring Philip back into the conversation. In effect, the therapist moves from a 'content' discussion to a 'process' discussion. In so doing, he highlights an awareness of the potential for the child to feel excluded by this 'gossiping' format of the interaction between himself and the parents. This re-inclusion is achieved by directly questioning Philip about his emotional response to hearing these negative evaluations. Thus, the therapist's tentative discourse here potentially invites 'corrections' in working towards an account that all family members can take up.

Because the maintenance and dynamic between different members of the family can be tricky, practitioners may use different strategies. The following section is an example of using hyperbole or extremity as another technique.

Alignment Through Extreme Case Formulation

The term 'extreme case formulation' (ECF) was first introduced by Pomerantz (1986) and is not a description of grammatical accuracy but represents the social action performed by a speaker. ECFs characteristically refer to their object in an extremely minimising or extremely maximising format (Sidnell, 2004). Whenever a speaker makes an assessment, in conversation analysis, a response to that assessment is made relevant such that the hearer is positioned as being required to agree or disagree with the assessment (Pomerantz, 1984). Typically, an agreement with the initial assessment to be heard as an agreement, it typically needs to be formulated as an upgrade. For example, if someone says, 'it's a nice day' as an evaluative first statement, to be heard as agreeing, the respondent might say 'yes, it's beautiful'.

In this simple example, beautiful is heard as an 'upgrade' of nice and so the overall social action of the response is understood as an agreement. The use of ECFs is therefore an extension of this principle but in the use of an extreme evaluation the response is heard as ironic rather than agreeing. For example, in response to 'it's a nice day' if someone said, 'yes, it's the most beautiful day I have ever experienced in my whole life', their statement is likely to be heard as ironic or sarcastic. When used in the context of family therapy, we found that the judicious use of extremity functioned to support or promote therapeutic alignment. In the following extract, the middle-aged female therapist is navigating a way to align or connect with her teenage male client.

Beech Clinic: Taken from Kiyimba (2020b, p. 7)

```
Therapist:    ↑I ca:n't understand why anybody would want to
              have their eyebrow pierced (.) OK?
(0.6)
Therapist:    ↑but then I belong to the days of the dinosaurs
Client:       mm
Therapist:    OK? Right,
```

The context of this data extract is that the client has been complaining that his parents were prohibiting him from having his eyebrow pierced, which he was claiming to be unreasonable. Initially, the therapist appears to align with the non-present parents by expressing a similar perspective 'I can't understand why anybody would want to have their eyebrow pieced'. Having made that statement, her potential disalignment with her client is apparent, and she works to repair that disalignment by using an ECF. In making an extreme claim about her age, 'I belong to the days of the dinosaurs' she makes relevant a potential reason for the difference of opinion with her client. When someone makes an extreme claim such as this, the hearer will usually make a statement in response that mitigates the extremity. The following data is a good example of this:

Example: Taken from Kiyimba (2020b, p. 10)

```
Therapist:   supposing it's all absolutely true ↑and you have
             got the meanest dad in the country
Client:      ↑Oh no he's not mean, he's just, well he can be
             he's jus' erm j's tight.
```

The ECF in this example is made by the therapist that the client may have the 'meanest dad in the country'. By placing an evaluation at an extreme end of the spectrum, this social action precipitates a more tempered response from the client. In this case, he responds by saying 'he's not mean' … 'he's jus' tight', which softens the meaning as tight is a colloquial expression for being careful with money.

Rupture

> **Rupture**
> Rupture is a technical term for when disalignment or a breakdown in the rapport occurs between the family member and the practitioner.

The term rupture is frequently used in counselling and therapy to denote a juncture in the professional conversation whereby there has been a breakdown or deterioration in the relationship between the client and practitioner (Safran & Muran, 1996). Ideally, this is something that practitioners try to avoid as much as possible, because the goals of the professional relationship are jeopardised. Ultimately, there is a potential that the family may completely disengage from services. However, in these instances, the practitioner can utilise skills to repair the rupture. There are multitudinous ways that rupture can happen in professional relationships, just as in ordinary interactions. They fall broadly into two categories, that of confrontation and withdrawal (Safran et al., 2001), and we argue that in the case of withdrawal, this can be passive or active. We focus on four types of rupture with examples from our data. These are inattention, disruption, resistance, and discontinuity.

Inattention

As noted in this chapter, the task for the practitioner of maintaining engagement with all family members requires skill and flexibility. It is very easy to engage in conversation with one family member and inadvertently exclude another family member. When inattention to a family member occurs, there could be a rupture in that dynamic. The following example is one where the therapist is in conversation with the father, and in doing so has for a period been inattentive to the child who is also present (taken from O'Reilly & Parker, 2013, p. 501).

Niles family

```
FT:       but it might be helpful,
Steve:    I'm ↓bored
FT:       for us t' at le:ast 'ave some ↑guesses about what's goin'
          on with Steve hhh so my kind of ↑first question is >what
          is it< [like (.) for you ↑Steve (0.2) sittin' 'ere =
Steve:           [I ↑wanna go 'ome
FT:       = hearin' us all talkin' about (0.2) the things that
          <you do> that are ↑naughty
```

The interaction proceeds with the therapist and father discussing the child Steve who is present. Steve's interjection 'I'm bored' and 'I wanna go 'ome' (as in, want to go home) is indicative of his disengagement from the process due to neither the father nor therapist maintaining engagement with him at that point. The therapist seeks to repair the rupture that has occurred by turning his attention to Steve 'what's it like for you Steve, sitting 'ere'. Typically, when a repair to rupture is initiated, the person being reincluded in the conversation will be addressed by their first name, which is 'Steve' in this example. Another good example of this can be found in the following extract (taken from O'Reilly & Parker,

2013, p. 497) where the child is re-engaged in the conversation by using his first name 'Bob'.

Bremner family

```
FT:     S::o Bob would you like [t' tell me why mummy's in a ↓mood
Bob:                             [No ↑I'm not in the mood ta tell
        (0.4) you
```

Disruption

When a practitioner has not attended to a particular family member (usually children) during a multi-party interaction, this may result in disengagement or boredom as described in the previous section. Furthermore, inattention may escalate into disruption whereby the unattended family member engages in behaviour to elicit attention or to lead to a termination of the interaction. We provide an example of this whereby two of the three children present begin to jump on the furniture (taken from O'Reilly & Parker, 2013, p. 496).

Clamp family

```
Dad:    I don't think Jordan understands what you're on about
        either (.) to be honest
FT:     Yeah
Dad:    I think Phil[lip(         )
Ron:               [Heh h[eh heh heh ((Ron is jumping))
Jordan:                  [heh heh heh heh ((Jordan is
        jumping))
Dad:    ↑Will you stop jumpin'
```

Because the therapist and the father have been talking without involving the children, there is a major rupture occurring in the session. Potentially, there may have been opportunities for the rupture to therapeutic alignment with the children to have been repaired at an earlier stage; however at this point, the disruptive behaviour of the children risks rupture of the whole session not just of alignment between one or two family members and the practitioner.

Notably, the two forms of rupture discussed, inattention and disruption, reflect the category of withdrawal proposed by Safran et al. (2001), with our first extract being an example of passive withdrawal and our second being active withdrawal. We now provide a form of rupture that is consistent with the notion of confrontation.

Resistance

With the examples we have illustrated, it can be easy for the adults to dominate the conversation. This may be unintentional and thus it is helpful for practitioners to be mindful of their decision about deliberate inclusion or exclusion of children in conversation with family members (which we return to later in the book). We invite our readers to be deliberate in their decision making about the inclusion or exclusion of children in conversations with families and to have a rationale for doing so. Where the decision has been made to include children in the interaction, it is important to ensure that therapeutic alignment is maintained with the children as well as adults. In circumstances where there has been a failure to attend to the importance of establishing and maintaining rapport with children, outright resistance may occur as is illustrated in the following example (taken from Parker & O'Reilly, 2013, p. 499).

Bremner family

```
FT:    ↑So (.) will you >come back again< (.) and see me again
       in fo:ur weeks?
Bob:   No
FT:    ↑Oh I think ↑so
Bob:   I will not
```

> If the decision has been taken to include children in the session, it is important to consistently engage them in the interaction to avoid rupture.

Discontinuity

Discontinuity can happen in various forms when working with families, and these can be broadly conceptualised into three types: expected, unexpected, and possible. Expected discontinuity refers to situations such as in family therapy where the therapist will routinely be expected to leave the room to consult with the reflecting team before returning to the family. Unexpected discontinuity refers to unplanned interruptions such as a knock on the door or telephone call or fire alarm sounding. Possible discontinuity refers to situations where there is a chance of unplanned disruption which can be anticipated and contingency measures put in place, such as arranging alternative communication modalities when engaged in online work. In the case of possible or unexpected discontinuity, there is likely to be a disruption to the flow of the interaction which may result in rupture. However, even in the case of planned discontinuity unless this is handled carefully, there may also be risk of therapeutic rupture. Ideally, the management of planned discontinuity would consist of three phases (the three P's of planned discontinuity):

1. *Pre-empting*—Signalling earlier in the session that a planned break in the session will occur.
2. *Performing*—Choosing the moment of discontinuity carefully and collaboratively agreeing the purpose and length.
3. *Picking up*—Re-entering the discontinued conversation by picking up where you left off.

The following series of extracts are examples of each of these phases in practice (taken from Parker & O'Reilly, 2013, p. 172).

Clamp family

```
FT:    Okay at some stage I might nip o:ut (.) jus' t' see if
       they've got any ideas, that might be helpful erm it gives
       you a bit [of space as well to think about (1.0) =
Dad:             [Yeah]
FT:    = or what you think about me and what we've been doing
```

Pre-empting

This extract is taken relatively from early on in a family therapy session. The therapist (FT) pre-empts that he may need to exit the session at some point to speak to the reflecting team. The key components of this pre-emption are beneficial to mitigating rupture and can be conceptualised in a four-part framework: stating that (a) it will occur (*'at some stage'*), (b) it will be brief (*'nip out'*), (c) the benefit to the therapist for the break (*'see if they've got any ideas'*), and (d) the potential benefit to the family for the break (*'gives you a bit of space as well'*). The following extract provides an example of performing an expected discontinuity break (taken from Parker & O'Reilly, 2013, p. 172).

Niles family

```
FT: In fact, (.) do yer want me t' leave you finishin' off that
    list if if >the two of you< do your ↑own list (.) which
    ones of those you think are like Steve (.) I'll go an'
    talk t' Carla (.) and I'll be back in a minute
```

> Whether the discontinuity is expected or possible, the benefits of pre-empting the interruption are that manages the expectations of the family members in a way that offers some protection against rupture.

Performing

Having prepared the family earlier in the session for the planned exit, the therapist now engages in performing that action. He does so by engaging in the latter three of the four components of the framework (b, c, and d) described previously: benefit to therapist ('go an' talk to Carla'), benefit to family ('do your own list'), and short timeframe ('back in a minute'). Engaging in each of these components does not take long but is an effective strategy in managing potential for rupture.

Picking up

The next extract is an example of picking up (taken from Parker & O'Reilly, 2013, p. 175).

Clamp family

```
FT:    Er::m (.) did you get chance to think a↑bout that
       question
       o::r (.) did you jus' ↓kind ↓of
Dad:   ↑I can't remember what it was n↑ow
FT:    Relax for a bit? (.)
Mum:   heh heh heh
FT:    don't worry about it (.) It was it it was ↑about (.) ↑I
       guess what you may have lea::rned from your dad about
       how t' be a dad (1.2) er::m (.) but that is a very hard
       question >I know< you may need more time to think about
       it (1.0) Er::m (1.0) I'll just I'll just say a little
       bit about er::m (.) what I was talkin' about with my (1.0)
       colleagues
```

Where expected and planned discontinuity is performed, the third component of re-entry to the conversation should be engaged in a way that creates an environment of continuity. This is achieved by picking up on the topic of conversation that was being discussed prior to the therapist exiting the room, upon re-entry ('did you get a chance to think about that question?'). In this way, the latter two parts of the framework (c and d) are invoked: the therapist orients to what was potentially beneficial to the family during that break ('what you may have learned from your dad'), before going onto discuss what was beneficial to the therapist during the break ('what I was talkin' about with my colleagues'). By maintaining coherence to the components of this simple four-part framework, even in an environment of discontinuity where rupture is a highly probable attention to these straightforward strategies can help to avoid that from happening. Notably, if the discontinuity is unexpected, then there will not have been an opportunity to pre-empt it beforehand, as in the case of expected or possible discontinuity.

Taking Responsibility for Rupture Management

We argue that there is an onus on the practitioner to hold some responsibility for recognising and predicting the possibility that rupture can occur in family interactions in several different ways. Practitioners can deliberately take steps to avoid rupture where possible and to develop skills to manage and repair rupture in situations where it is unavoidable. When working with families, it is a complex task for practitioners to maintain active engagement with all family members consistently. There is a challenge to maintain active engagement of children in part due to their membership status and in part due to their developmental competence and attention span. We have illustrated in this section of the chapter, some of the ways that children can be marginalised or disengaged from the therapeutic conversations. These were inattention, disruption, and resistance. Where children have temporarily disengagement, re-engagement can be achieved by using their first name, asking them direct questions, encouraging them to reflect on things, and sharing their own perspectives. Another point made was that validating the child's experience both outside the current interaction and in the here and now listening to the conversations between the adult parties is a powerful way of maintaining children's engagement. Acknowledging and validating the challenges for the child in the current interaction, such as becoming bored, hearing negative appraisals about their behaviour, and potential uncertainties they face, can create space for them to feel more accepted. In some ways, this resonates with mentalisation-based treatments in family therapy (Hantel-Quitmann & Weidtmann, 2016). To consolidate your thinking about this section of the chapter, we invite you to engage with the reflective activity in Box 3.1.

> **Box 3.1 Reflective Activity on Rupture**
>
> Reflective activity
> Rupture
> Based on what you have read in this section of the chapter, we invite you to reflect on the questions below to think about your own practice in avoiding, managing, and repairing rupture when working with families:
>
> 1. What strategies do you currently have in place to manage and repair rupture?
> 2. How do you intentionally plan to avoid rupture?
> 3. How do you actively engage children in conversations with families?
> 4. How might shorter sessions potentially avoid children's boredom, disruption, and disengagement?
> 5. What environmental considerations could you consider that might support consistent engagement with all family members?

Interruptions

The Western cultural norm in social interaction is that there is a turn-taking process whereby one speaker takes the conversational floor at a time. Normatively, the social etiquette in conversation is that one speaker speaks at a time and the listener waits for the current speaker to conclude their turn before speaking. Thus, the moment-by-moment allocation of turns is a social accomplishment (Lerner, 1989). This social accomplishment is guided by the norms of society and is a small part of the larger social accomplishment of normative practices of appropriate behaviour. As with any social construct of normative action, there is a need for much of a particular society to agree on specific norms as being preferable. Turn taking in conversation is an example of a socially constructed social norm for social interaction, and thus is an interactional accomplishment. For children in families, it is part of their developmental socialisation that parents and other adults will instruct them in the art of turn-taking.

Interrupting is a way of describing a breach of the social norm of conversational turn-taking. In conversation analysis, the terminology used is 'the conversational floor', which refers to the space people occupy when they are taking turns in a conversation. In other words, it is a usual practice for one person to speak while the other listens, and then change speaker at an appropriate moment. The speaker who is at any time speaking is the person who is holding the conversational floor. In multi-party conversations, like those with families, there may be competition for who is allocated or who initiates moving into that space of being the speaker and holding the conversational floor.

Conversation analysts have identified that typically listeners can recognise appropriate points when a speaker has completed their turn and it is relevant to provide a response. These transition points between one speaker's turn and the next speaker's turn are called Transition Relevance Places (TRPs) (Sacks et al., 1974). Notably, this is a sophisticated socio-discursive skill, and there are occasions in conversation where the listener misjudges the closing point of the speaker's turn and begins their turn. In this case, there is some overlapping talk, but this does not constitute an interruption (Jefferson, 1986). An interruption is when the second speaker begins a turn when there is no indication of a TRP or no TRP.

Power and Asymmetry

Different researchers subscribe to different ideas about the existence of power depending on their theoretical framework. Although this is a complex epistemological issue, broadly speaking from a macro-social constructionism position, power exists and is a concept that is used as a presupposition, whereas from a micro-social constructionist position, power does not pre-exist before it is co-created between members. Many feminist researchers also approach research from the starting point that power pre-exists a social interaction. Feminists have been influential in the study of interruptions because of their viewpoint that there are power differentials between men and women, and conversational interruptions are the only mechanism by which this power is realised (Fishman, 1983; Lakoff, 1990; West & Zimmerman, 1983). This is because an interruption intrusively disrupts the speaker's turn and by implication the interrupter is asserting dominance over the speaker (Zimmerman & West, 1975).

The feminist and macro-social constructionist perspective articulates conversational interruptions as performing a social action of invocation of power and dominance. That is, they have an *a priori* assumption that an interruption always represents the social action of dominance. However, our preference for approaching data inductively is to examine the social actions accomplished by interruptions by examining actual family interactions in situ. This micro-social constructionist approach views interruptions as a discursive action without pre-assuming the existence of power. Additionally, we concur with Hutchby (1992) who argues that the attribution of a discursive action as an interruption is an evaluative construct achieved by the members of the social interaction. In other words, treating something as an interruption is an interpretation made by family members engaged in that specific conversation rather than being independently so. To do so, we analyse the way that participants orient to seemingly anomalous turns as potential social deviations to the turn-taking rule, or not.

Members Interrupting: Children

In the data we present, we consider the interactional accomplishments achieved when practitioners, parents, or children initiate a turn (take the conversational floor) during an ongoing turn of talk by another speaker (see also O'Reilly, 2006, 2008). We start by presenting two identifiably different types of interruptions initiated by children, (1) contextually non-relevant and (2) contextually relevant, to the institutional business of therapy. In response to the contextually non-relevant interruptions, there were two types of responses from the adults, which were either to ignore the child or to reprimand them. In response to contextually relevant interruptions, typically the child was engaged in the conversation.

Here, we present two examples of contextually non-relevant interruptions from children. The first is where the child interrupts his father and the second is where the child interrupts the practitioner. In both cases, the child is ignored.

Clamp family (taken from O'Reilly, 2006, p. 554)

```
Dad:      Ronald's okay n↑o[w then Ron↓ald ain't too ↓bad =
→Phil:                [°Can I play with Jordan dad?°
Dad:      = >I mean< 'e 'as be'aviour problems >sometimes< but.
          'e's just (.) >you know< .hh it's <↑not the same
          a:s> (.)
          whatev↓er
FT:       Ye↓ah
```

Bremner family (taken from O'Reilly, 2006, p. 557)

```
Gran:     No °no°
FT:       ↑No not at [this moment
→Bob:                [Pick a num↑ber
FT:       I've just se:en the time (0.4) the time's flown by
Gran:     Yea::h
```

In the first extract, the father is talking with the practitioner about his son Ronald's behaviour and his other son Philip interrupts to ask his father a question 'can I play with Jordan dad?'. The child's interruption is not related to the institutional business of the conversation between his father and the practitioner and is therefore categorised as 'contextually non-relevant'. The father does not acknowledge the question or respond to it, and thus in effect ignores this interruptive question. In the second extract, the practitioner is in conversation with the grandmother and the child, Bob, interrupts by asking the practitioner to join his game by selecting a number in a 'pick a number' game. Again, this is an example of a child's interruption that is contextually non-relevant and like the first example is ignored by the adult parties. The following extract is an example of the second kind of response to contextually non-relevant interruptions by a child where instead of being ignored, the child is reprimanded.

Niles family (taken from O'Reilly, 2006, p. 559/60)

```
FT:    ↑but then ↑Steve >didn't want to know< (.) he was kind of
       no way >leave me alone< hh ↑bu[t then when you =
Lee:                                 [°I want Joe°
FT:    = went back he told you
Dad:   Oi (0.2) shut up.
FT:    When you're u[pset Nicky, what do you like pe:ople to =
Lee:                [I want to talk to Joe
FT:    =do (0.4) if you'[re upset >what do you like people to do<
Dad:                    [He'll talk to you in a minute when he's
       finished
```

At this point in the interaction, the practitioner and the parents are conversing about the oldest son's problematic behaviour. This topic of conversation is contextually relevant to the institutional business of therapy. When the child interrupts this conversation twice with an apparently contextually non-relevant request for attention from the therapist 'I want Joe' and 'I want to talk to Joe', his father reprimands him on both occasions for the interruption. It is clear from the father's response to the child's request that he treats it as a breach of social interaction rules. The father tells the child to stop talking 'shut up' and to have patience, 'he'll talk to you in a minute'.

The previous examples have illustrated two kinds of adult responses to children's interruptions that were categorised as 'contextually non-relevant'. We now look at an example from an interaction where a child interrupts the adult speakers with what we refer to as a 'contextually relevant' comment. In other words, although the child does not wait for someone to finish speaking before speaking themselves, the topic of what they are saying is relevant to the topic of the conversation between the adults.

Niles family (taken from O'Reilly, 2006, p. 562)

```
Mum:     And 'e got 'is hair off with that and >chucked it< on
         the flo::or >and I says< we[ll once ↓yo-
Steve:                              [NO I HAVEn't I dropped *it
         on the ↑flo:or
Dad:     <YOU [threw it> across the livin' ro:om befo:re n↑ow
Mum:          [N- <YOU CHUCKED IT> .hh I was ↑there and seen ya
         >and I says< once you break that <you ARE NOT 'avin'
         another one> because they're not ↓cheap they are a lot
         of money.
```

Here, we see the mother describing the child's bad behaviour, with 'got his hair off'. This being an English colloquial phrase to mean losing one's temper. The mother states that her son 'chucked' something onto the floor, at which point he interrupts her turn to counter her claim by arguing that he 'dropped it'. This extract is an example of a child's interruption that is contextually relevant in the sense that it is part of the ongoing conversation about the child's behaviour. Arguably what this extract is an example of, is the fact that adults respond to a child's interruption if it is contextually relevant to the institutional business, whereas the previous extracts showed that interruptions that were not aligned with the content of the conversation or topic were ignored or dismissed. The success or failure of a child's attempt to take the conversational floor appears to rely on their interactional competence to judge the appropriateness or relevance of an interjection as it pertains to the institutional business set by the adult parties.

Members Interrupting: Practitioners

In addition to investigating children's interruptions, we also looked at practitioner interruptions of adult family members' talk. Notably, the data in our research indicated that the turn construction of practitioners' interruptions was characterised by politeness markers, which were absent in the children's interruptions. In terms of social competence, politeness markers are displays of attending to social schemas. Social schemas are normative patterns of behaviours that are expected in different contexts, for example, how to behave in a restaurant or what is normatively

3 Forming and Maintaining Good Relationships

expected of people in a classroom setting. In relation to politeness, a social schema is a framework within a cultural context of what behaviours are deemed to be polite or impolite. In the data we have presented, the social schema for that cultural context is that it is impolite to interrupt someone while they are speaking, and it is polite to wait for that person to finish speaking before you start your own turn of talk. In our data, when practitioners did interrupt adult family members, they did so by orienting to the shared cultural understanding that it was as a rule, impolite to interrupt. The way this is managed interactionally is to say something that indicates an apology for the social breach, at the same time as engaging in that social breach. In this case, the social breach was to interrupt someone whilst they are speaking. The form of apology for that interruption is called a 'politeness marker' in discourse analysis terms. However, there was a clear differentiation between the use of politeness markers when practitioners interrupted adults, compared to a lack of politeness markers when practitioners interrupted children.

A phrase that has been used to describe the rights of children compared to adults in multi-party, multi-generational conversation is that of 'half-membership' (see Hutchby & O'Reilly, 2010; Shakespeare, 1998). This refers to the constructed membership of certain population groups to hold interactional and social competencies to contribute to the ongoing conversation. Thus, membership status refers to the ethos of equality with all members having equal participation rights with children being encouraged to engage and be included, but because of developmental and social competencies, children are often treated as having less interactional rights than their adult counterparts (Hutchby & O'Reilly, 2010). The following two examples illustrate the orientation of the practitioner to a self-awareness of making an interruptive turn.

Niles family (taken from O'Reilly, 2008, p. 512)

```
Mrs Niles:  >I mean< I did, suggest when I [went to se:e
            that doc↓tor
FT:                                        [>Can I ↑just< say
            as well, sorry (.) <sorry to interrupt> (.) i- if
            this is <about Steve> kind of (.) struggling with
            *stuff ↑emotionally .hh that doesn't me::an that
            you're doin' a bad. j↓ob.
```

Clamp family (taken from O'Reilly, 2008, p. 513)

```
Mr Clamp:   re:ally they're sayin' that Joe's done s[omethin'
            ↓right,
FT:                                                  [w- w- w-
            >can I< <can> (.) I I know I'm ↑interruptin' 'ere
            Dan, and I'm ↑sorry [about that, (.) it's e::rm
Mr Clamp:                       [No you're al↑ri:ght
```

Both examples show that the practitioner is reflexively aware that the social action is an interruption and is therefore accountable (meaning that if you do something that breaches normal social convention, you would be expected to give an account or explanation for doing so). Rather than not interrupting, they maintain the interruption and mitigate it via an apology. This convention is contrasted with the following two examples whereby the practitioner interrupts a child without recourse to any social conventions such as an apology.

Niles family (taken from O'Reilly, 2008, p. 517)

```
FT:      ↑Ah you watch it as well >do you< Steve?
Steve:   ↓No
Lee:     >He does we a[ll< °watch-°
FT:                   [How do you know that Bart's naughty?
```

Bremner family (taken from O'Reilly, 2008, p. 518)

```
Gran:   ↑Oh ↑right (.) ↓yeah
Bob:    And I was go[in' to s-
FT:                 [So unfortunately <sorry I had to cancel>
        the appointment 'cause I was unwell.
```

In the first of these two examples, the practitioner is addressing the child Lee's brother, Steve, to ask about whether the family watches the television show, *The Simpsons* (a topic we return to again later in the book). After, Steve's negative response, Lee takes his turn at an appropriate transition relevance place, to make a comment that is contextually relevant to the conversation 'we all watch'. However, the practitioner seemingly ignores Lee's contribution and interrupts his attempt to offer a different perspective. In the second example, the child, Bob, starts to make a statement 'I was goin' to' but is interrupted by the practitioner before he can complete his turn. Again, the practitioner seemingly ignores the child's interjection. The turn initial marker 'so' is indicative of a topic shift or advancing the interactional agenda (Bolden, 2009) and demonstrates that the practitioner makes a conversational move that is apparently not client- or child-centred.

We are mindful here that this analysis may ostensibly appear critical of practice; however, these examples are not unusual and are representative of many institutional and mundane settings whereby adult members are conversing with populations conceived to have half membership. When children interrupt conversations, it may be that their developmental competence in social interaction is not as sophisticated as adults and they inadvertently miss transition relevance places and/or are not sufficiently aware of the contextual relevance and/or all family members are caught up in an unquestioned pattern of interaction. We invite the reader to consider that although children's attempts to engage in an adult interaction may not always be interactionally suitable, their contributions could be viewed as ways to try to be involved. As such, practitioners may find it helpful to be aware of this in intergenerational professional conversations.

Final Thoughts

The overarching theme of this chapter has been the importance and potential fragility of the relational alignment between different members of the family and the practitioner. Within this, we have used data to explore the ways in which therapeutic relationships are developed, maintained, and repaired. Specifically, we have explored some potential junctures at which therapeutic rupture may occur and how this can be avoided or repaired. We argue that responsibility for anticipating potential rupture and making an effort to manage it lies predominantly with the practitioner. Finally, we have presented some interesting observations about the difference between the ways in which child and adult interruptions are treated in institutional contexts. As we bring this chapter to a close, we offer the insights of a clinical practitioner, Dr Philip Archard, who works with families daily regarding the value of the messages and reflexive considerations generated from this chapter. These thoughts are outlined in Box 3.2.

Box 3.2 Practitioner Voice, Philip Archard

Practitioner voices
Dr Philip Archard
Mental health practitioner in CAMHS

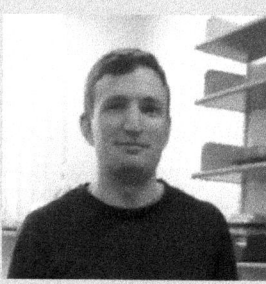

Dr Philip Archard is mental health practitioner working in the child and adolescent mental health service of Leicestershire Partnership NHS Trust. Outside of his clinical work, he is active in research and an honorary associate professor at the University of Leicester and a visiting lecturer at the Tavistock and Portman NHS Foundation Trust.

I practice in a specialist child and adolescent mental health service team serving children from various groups considered vulnerable to a high level of mental health need, including children who living in residential or foster care, who are adopted, who are unaccompanied asylum seekers, and who are involved with the criminal justice system. My role is a generic position that can be filled by different healthcare professions (most often, social workers, mental health nurses, psychologists, or occupational therapists). I came to this role with some background in applied social science alongside my core professional training, meaning I view the work via something of a combination of psychodynamic and sociological lenses.

The work is challenging—one needs to turn one's hand to a range of different tasks: care coordination and attendance at multiagency forums and meetings, as well as individual therapy, consultation and training for parents and professional carers, and general and specialised assessments. All these tasks are done against quite significant time constraints and with a heavy workload—I often find myself fantasising about stepping away from the fray to return to the role of ethnographer. At the same time, there is much to learn in the doing of the work, and, for me, the therapeutic relationship (or some notion of it) is something that can be both under- and over-estimated by clinicians. On the one hand, the well-worn trope of the importance of the child–clinician relationship beyond the therapeutic

(continued)

> **Box 3.2 (continued)**
>
> modality practised is something I hear oft repeated. On the other hand (and perhaps partly why it seems so crucial yet also misunderstood), pressures of service demand mean that relationships with children, young people, and their families are often short-lived, and insufficient time is available to work through ruptures or breakdowns that are more likely when working with the socially marginalised groups my team serves.
>
> Reviewing this chapter led me to think a lot about children's voices and how they are implicitly conceptualised in the field of child and adolescent mental health, particularly at the interface between mental health and child welfare services. I would agree that it is easy to overlook how apparent disruptions or disturbances by children in conversations involving carers and families can signal a desire to be involved in a conversation—albeit the overlooking of this can often, I find, have something to do emotional intensity of these conversations and the extent of the distress being experienced. Equally, what is viewed as being in a child's best interests regarding their mental health by involved adults (family, carers, and professionals) can be conflated with what is best for them more generally, serving to omit their voice from discussions about how they might be helped and what they need to be helped with—even, it may be said, negating their role as agentic subjects. At its most basic, for me, this reinforces the need to continue to work at being a good listener, in terms of how clinical encounters unfold and interactions are managed by those present, but also to decipher and translate the different personal, professional, and organisational investments underlying what is said and communicated.

On reflection of this chapter, it is evident how sophisticated family conversations are in terms of the nuances of turn-taking practices that are inherently learned through the process of development and socialisation into a certain culture. It is often only at the point of rupture or disalignment that these otherwise seamless turn-taking practices occur. An added layer of complexity to the social conventions of normative conversational interaction is when there is a specific institutional agenda. The efforts of children to contribute to multi-party intergenerational interactions in an institutional interaction demonstrate the high level of social competence required to achieve this successfully. Through writing this chapter and reflecting on the data, we are reminded that maintaining strongly aligned relationships with all family members is a challenging and difficult endeavour. Yet it is with frameworks of child-centredness and the

> **Box 3.3 Key Points**
>
> - Research indicates that the strength of a therapeutic relationship is integral to success of any family intervention.
> - Three ways that alignment can be achieved in institutional interactions is via active listening, re-inclusion of any talked about third party, and the ironic use of extreme formulations to alleviate tensions.
> - Rupture in the relationship can have important consequences such as disengagement from services.
> - Children's inattention, disruption, or resistance during family interventions may indicate attempts to be involved in the conversation.
> - Practitioner's use of interruptions to navigate the conversation to institutional business can be achieved through politeness markers and orientation to this action as accountable.
> - There may be benefit in reflecting on the function of children's interruptions and what they might be trying to communicate.

importance of engagement for strong outcomes, practitioners benefit from working with the evidence base and sharing examples of good practice. To conclude, therefore, we direct the reader to the summary key points in Box 3.3.

References

Anderson, H. (2001). Postmodern collaborative and person-centred therapies: What would Carl Rogers say? *Journal of Family Therapy, 23*(4), 339–360.

Atkinson, D., Churchill, E., Nishino, T., & Okada, H. (2007). Alignment and interaction in a sociocognitive approach to second language acquisition. *Modern Language Journal, 91*, 169–188.

Bolden, G. (2009). Implementing incipient actions: The discourse marker 'so' in English conversation. *Journal of Pragmaticis, 45*, 974–998.

DeAngelis, T. (2019). Better relationships with patients lead to better outcomes. *American Psychological Association, 50*(10), 38. retrieved from https://www.apa.org/monitor/2019/11/ce-corner-relationships

DiFonzo, N., & Bordia, P. (2007). Rumor, gossip, and urban legends. *Diogenes, 213*, 19–35.

Fishman, P. (1983). Interaction: The work women do. In B. Thorne, C. Kramarae, & N. Henley (Eds.), *Language, gender, and society* (pp. 89–101). Newbury House.

Foster, E. (2004). Research on gossip: Taxonomy, methods, and future directions. *Review of General Psychology, 8*(2), 78–99.

Geldard, K., & Geldard, D. (1998). *Counselling children: A practical introduction*. Sage.

Hantel-Quitmann, W., & Weidtmann, K. (2016). Family climate, parental partner relationships and symptom formation in children-mentalisation-based family therapy for childhood headache. *Praxis der Kinderpsychologie und Kinderpsychiatrie, 65*(1), 22–39.

Hutchby, I. (2005). "Active Listening": Formulations and the elicitation of feelings-talk in child counselling. *Research on Language and Social Interaction, 38*, 303–329.

Hutchby, I. (1992). Confrontation talk: Aspects of 'Interruption' in argument sequences on talk radio. *Text, 12*(3), 343–371.

Hutchby, I., & O'Reilly, M. (2010). Children's participation and the familial moral order in family therapy. *Discourse Studies, 12*(1), 49–64.

Jefferson, G. (1986). Notes on latency in overlap onset. *Human Studies, 9*, 153–183.

Kiyimba, N. (2020a). *Trauma-informed mindfulness: A Practitioner's guide for one-to-one work*. University of Chester.

Kiyimba, N. (2020b). 'I belong to the days of the dinosaurs': Extreme case formulation in therapeutic practice. *Qualitative Psychology, 7*(3), 384–397.

Lakoff, R. (1990). *Talking power: The politics of language in our lives*. Basic Books.

Lambert, M., & Barley, D. (2001). Research summary on the therapeutic relationship and psychotherapy outcome. *Psychotherapy: Theory, Research, Practice Training, 38*(4), 357–361.

Lerner, G. (1989). Notes on overlap Management in Conversation: The case of delayed completion. *Western Journal of Speech Communication., 53*, 167–177.

Michelson, G., van Iterson, A., & Waddington, K. (2010). Gossip in organisations: Contexts, consequence, and controversies. *Group & Organization Management, 35*(4), 371–390.

Nofsinger, R. (1991). *Everyday conversation*. Sage.

Noon, M., & Delbridge, R. (1993). News from behind my hand: Gossip in organizations. *Organization Studies, 14*(1), 23–36.

Ohta, A. (2001). From acknowledgment to alignment: A longitudinal study of the development of expression of alignment by classroom learners of Japanese. In G. Kasper & K. Rose (Eds.), *Pragmatics in language teaching* (pp. 103–120). University Press.

O'Reilly, M. (2006). Should children be seen and not heard? An examination of how children's interruptions are treated in family therapy. *Discourse Studies, 8*(4), 549–566.

O'Reilly, M. (2008). 'What value is there in children's talk?' Investigating family therapist's interruptions of parents and children during the therapeutic process. *Journal of Pragmatics, 40*, 507–524.

O'Reilly, M., & Parker, N. (2013). 'You can take a horse to water but you can't make it drink': Exploring children's engagement and resistance in family therapy. *Contemporary Family Therapy, 35*(3), 491–507.

Parker, N., & O'Reilly, M. (2013). Reflections from behind the screen: Avoiding therapeutic rupture when utilising reflecting teams. *The Family Journal: Counseling for Couples and Families, 21*(2), 170–179.

Parker, N., & O'Reilly, M. (2012). 'Gossiping' as a social action in family therapy: The pseudo-absence and pseudo-presence of children. *Discourse Studies, 14*(4), 1–19.

Peräkylä, A. (1995). *AIDS counselling: Institutional interaction and clinical practice*. Cambridge University Press.

Pomerantz, A. (1986). Extreme case formulations: A way of legitimizing claims. *Human Studies, 9*(2–3), 219–229.

Pomerantz, A. (1984). Agreeing and disagreeing with assessments: Some features of preferred/dispreferred turn shapes. In J. Atkinson & J. Heritage (Eds.), *Structures of social action: Studies in conversation analysis* (pp. 57–101). Cambridge University Press.

Rogers, C. (1957). The necessary and sufficient conditions of therapeutic personality change. *Journal of Consulting Psychology, 21*(2), 95.

Sacks, H., Schegloff, E., & Jefferson, G. (1974). A simplest systematics for the organization of turn-taking for conversation. *Language, 50*(4), 696–735.

Safran, J., & Muran, C. (1996). The resolution of ruptures in the therapeutic alliance. *Journal of Consulting and Clinical Psychology, 64*(3), 447–458.

Safran, J., Muran, C., Samstag, L., & Stevens, C. (2001). Repairing alliance ruptures. *Psychotherapy, 38*(4), 406–412.

Sidnell, J. (2004). There's risks in everything: Extreme-case formulations and accountability in inquiry testimony. *Discourse & Society, 15*, 745–766.

Shakespeare, P. (1998). *Aspects of confused speech: A study of verbal interaction between confused and normal speakers*. Lawrence Erlbaum Associates.

Spencer-Oatey, H. (Ed.). (2004). *Culturally speaking: Managing rapport through talk across cultures*. A&C Black.

Spencer-Oatey, H., & Žegerac, V. (2017). Power, solidarity and (im)politeness. In J. Culpeper, M. Haugh, & D. Z. Kádár (Eds.), *The Palgrave handbook of linguistic (im)politeness* (pp. 119–141). Basingstoke: Palgrave.

Tecedor, M. (2016). Beginning Learners' development of interactional competence: Alignment activity. *Foreign Language Annals, 49*(1), 23–41.

West, C., & Zimmerman, D. (1983). Small insults: A study of Interruptions in cross-sex conversations with unacquainted persons. In B. Thorne, C. Kramarae & N. Henley (Eds), *Language, gender and society* (pp. 102–117). Rowley: Newbury House.

Zimmerman, D., & West, C. (1975). Sex roles, interruptions and silences in conversations. In B. Thorne & N. Henley (Eds.), *Language and sex: Difference and dominance* (pp. 225–274). Newbury House.

Part II

Engaging Children

4

Designing Questions with Children

Learning Objectives

- Recognise the importance of question design
- Critically assess different ways of engaging children in mental health interactions
- Identify ways to ask a question to elicit elaborated answers from children
- Reflect on different questioning styles and techniques

Introduction

Engaging children and young people in service interactions is a crucial part of mental health business. In mental health interactions, such as child counselling, family therapy, mental health assessments and so on, there is an institutional assumption that the client will engage and comply with the service expectations (Silverman, 1997). To engage children in these endeavours, practitioners have become more child-centred, recognising the value of children's contributions (Dogra, 2005). This child-centred ideology is congruent with the wider treaty of children's rights (United Nations, 1989). That is, the global initiative for all countries who are signed up to take seriously the rights of children to be actively involved in decisions that affect them. Healthcare services operationalise this treaty through their care pathways and their commitment to communicate with and fully engage children in all aspects of their mental health appointment. In this chapter, we offer evidence-based recommendations and practical ideas for practitioners to effectively communicate with, and engage, children in conversations that relate to their healthcare.

The Value of Questions and the Importance of Question Design

It is important in institutional discourse to understand question and answer sequences (Ehrlich & Freed, 2010), because these are central to the institutional business and perform a range of different functions (James et al., 2010). For example, in the context of assessing mental health, questions primarily function to elicit sufficient information to make a reliable diagnosis (Thompson & McCabe, 2016). Rather than critically examining practitioners' question design as the potential reason for misalignment, non-engagement or therapeutic rupture, previous research suggests that some practitioners misattribute poor clinical outcomes to client resistance and avoidance (James et al., 2010).

To properly evaluate the form and function of questions in situ, there is great value in drawing upon recordings of actual healthcare interactions. As we noted earlier in the book, our naturally occurring data is a rich and in-depth source for analysing question design in practice. By interrogating real-world practices and exploring question use in context, we can learn valuable lessons about effective question design and placement. The effectiveness of a question is not merely the form that the questions take but also the situated use of that question within the institutional context, the way in which the question is asked and its intonation (Kiyimba et al., 2017).

Working closely in clinical academic partnerships to analyse and reflect on the role of questions in mental health settings, we have come to recognise the valuable role that well-formed and well-placed questions can have in allowing children and young people to fully articulate the aetiology, nature, and consequences of their difficulties. Careful design of the questions used and a reflective, engaging style can transform what might otherwise feel like a barrage of interrogation into a collaborative, facilitative dialogue.

Different Ways of Using Questions

Although the speech act of a question has particular grammatical features, questions vary considerably in the way that they are designed and the purposes for which they are employed. In the context of working with families, some questions asked by practitioners may be purely information seeking for institutional purposes, and other questions are therapeutically designed. An example of questions for therapeutic purposes are those used in interventive interviewing which are designed to facilitate reflective thinking on the part of the client (Tomm, 1987a, 1987b). Another example is the motivational interviewing approach whereby clients are enabled to resolve ambivalence and move forward on the readiness for change pathway using questions that elicit the client's own motives for change (Hettema et al., 2005).

Evidently, the design of a question is important for working with families, as the wording and agenda of the question will shape the answer. For example, some kinds of questions will specify a very narrow focus for answers, whereas others will provide opportunity for greater elaboration. From our data corpus we now present five domains of using questions that we have identified and explain their value for different purposes.

Closed Questions

These are also called interrogative or polar questions, as they typically invite a 'yes' or a 'no' response from the recipient. Contrary to some opinion, closed questions can be very useful, especially early on in an interaction, if a concrete response is required, and to help gather some foundational information. Closed questions can be used in question sequences initially to provide a basis for an open question when further detail is needed. We provide two examples of closed questions from our family mental health assessment data (taken from O'Reilly et al., 2015, p. 117).

Family 9

```
MHC    do you have any friends at school?
Child  yeah
```

Family 8

```
MHC    is that every day that something happens in school?
Child  ((child shakes head))
```

One of the especially valuable aspects of a closed question is that they do not tend to contain presuppositions or assumptions, and thus, either answer yes or no is equally acceptable. They function to check some factual basis prior to asking more exploratory questions related to that topic. Indeed, the subsequent questions will be designed differently and pursue different matters depending on the answer to the initial closed question. If we consider our example, 'do you have any friends?', if the child says yes, then open questions about those relationships can be asked, but if the child says no, then the potential for rupture is avoided from a possible assumption that the child does have friendships in school.

Wh-Prefaced Questions

Wh-prefaced questions consist of those questions that start with, *who*, *wh*at, *wh*ere, *wh*y, *wh*en, *wh*ich, and also 'how' (with how fitting the classification by its function rather than specifically starting 'wh'). Typically, wh-prefaced questions are open questions and generally pursue additional detail from the recipient. We provide examples below (taken from O'Reilly et al., 2015, p. 118).

Family 20

```
Prac   Which school are you going to?
Child  ((names school))
```

Family 1

```
Prac   how often do you do the touching?
Child  erm quite often like when I'm sorting my clothes out
       and that.
```

These are two simple examples of wh-prefaced questions in practice, illustrating that when seeking information or details, such questions work well to elicit answers. Although why questions are part of this classification, we have observed they do not always work as well, because of the implicit accountability that is embedded (Kiyimba et al., 2017). The extract below is a good example of this (taken from O'Reilly et al., 2015, p. 118).

Family 16

```
Prac   why do you take that?
Child  I don't know
```

Arguably, there is an inherent negativity embedded in a why question that implies that the content of the question is 'wrong' or inappropriate in some way. This is seen in the previous extract with the simple question 'why do you take that?'. It is hearable that the 'take that' is not something that should be done, simply by being prefaced by a question starting with 'why'. When we refer to embedded accountability, we mean that a question that implies some inappropriateness may require a justification, excuse, or rationale for the behaviour in response. The next extract (taken from Kiyimba et al., 2017, p. 234) is also a why question; however, aside from the implied accountability, there is also a presupposition made by the psychiatrist that the child (Kolomban) wanted to burn down the mother's bedroom.

Family 16

```
Mother  Kolomban wanted to ↓burn down my bedroom
Psych   °Right° (0.38) °why did you want to do that K↓olomban?°
Child   °I did↓n't
```

The child actively disagrees with the presupposition, by stating 'I didn't' demonstrating the risks of using wh-prefaced open questions before agreement has been reached about the underlying premise. The child is not disputing the fact that he started a fire in the bedroom, he is disputing the claim his mother makes that he *wanted to*. The psychiatrist's question demonstrates alignment with the mother's version of events without having established the child's perspective.

Declarative Questions

> **Declarative Question**
> This is a question that makes a statement but is delivered with a questioning tone.

Different practitioner disciplines may use different terminology to describe declarative questions. For example, in counselling and psychotherapy, these kinds of questions are often formulated as reflected statements that are offered back to the client with questioning intonation. Declarative questions tend to have a slight bias in the kinds of answers they provoke, which are usually affirmative. In other words, the recipient typically agrees with the statement offered through the question, whether positive or negative. In conversation analysis, this is referred to as 'preference organisation' (Bilmes, 1988). We provide three examples of these for illustrative purposes (examples from family 1 and family 2 taken from O'Reilly et al., 2015, p. 118; example from family 11 taken from O'Reilly et al., 2020, p. 556).

Family 1

```
Prac    but that time with your sister you did get the images?
Child   yeah
```

Family 2

```
Prac    so it wasn't the best day?
Child   ((child shakes head))
```

Family 11

```
Psych    >Okay so y- you didn't have (.) noth- nothing was
         ↓men[tioned]< (0.30)
Mother        [No no]
Psych    in terms of (.) ↓like (.) developmental ↓milestones,
         teething: (0.43) sitting (0.61) walking?
Mother   Everything was ↑normal [like a ↓normal] child ↑yeah
```

It seems that declarative questions perform three helpful functions simultaneously which can be beneficial when working with families:

1. They demonstrate active listening.
2. They check the accuracy of a shared understanding.
3. They provide an opportunity for elaboration and further discussion.

> **Tag Question**
> A short question that is 'tagged' onto the end of a statement, often seeking confirmation or refutation.

Where declarative questions are defined as a statement produced with questioning intonation, a tag question occurs where a statement is made with final or continuing intonation, and then a short question is 'tagged' at the end to transform it from a statement to a question (Thompson & McCabe, 2016). We provide two examples of tag questions to illustrate what they look like (taken from O'Reilly et al., 2015, p. 118).

Family 9

```
Prac     it's amazing when you've got loads of them. Isn't it?
Mother   yeah
```

Family 18

```
Prac     he only comes at the weekends did you say?
Child    yeah
```

Tag questions check the correctness of the statement made and are typically closed questions. These kinds of questions tend to perform a confirmation-seeking function and mostly acquire affirmative answers from the recipient. In practice, these kinds of questions can be useful when the practitioner is summarising and reflecting back a segment of information to the family and interjects tag questions throughout the summary to check the accuracy of the formulations offered.

> Short closed 'tag questions' can be added to statements to check their accuracy.

Either/Or Questions

Either/or questions are those that utilise the lexical item 'or' within the question to offer alternative possible answers for the recipient. Sometimes either/or questions can stipulate specific alternatives to a question, such as 'would you like a banana or an apple?'. In this example, the option of a bag of chips is not available. This use of an either/or question can be valuable when there is a benefit to maintaining some boundaries whilst also offering the client a degree of choice. Other examples might be 'would you like another appointment next Tuesday or Wednesday?'; 'would you prefer me to contact you by text or email?'. Other kinds of either/or questions might indicate the parameters or scope of the kind of answers that are appropriate without limiting the recipient too specifically. We provide an example (from Antaki & O'Reilly, 2014, p. 335). In this extract, the first part offered by the practitioner is reasonable, but the second part is more extreme.

Family 1

```
Prac    when you first sent her to: the nursery school,
Mum     yeah-
Prac    did she go ok: or (.) was there [a (big c]eremony
                       about       [it)]
                  Mum              [er ]
                                   [yeah sh]e cri:ed
```

Thus, the use of this continuum type of either/or question with an extreme option at one end 'a big ceremony' provides a spectrum of what might be deemed expected or appropriate responses. As we can see from the mother's response, she gives an answer that sits somewhere in the middle of the continuum of options for a child's first day at nursery school, 'yeah, she cried'. In practice, using either/or questions with extreme options can give permission for the family members to provide any kind of response or disclosure between those two extremities.

Summarising Thoughts

In writing about these domains of questions, we recognise that this is only a small set of examples of the many different types of question design. Practitioners working within the field of talking therapy may have a wide vocabulary of usage of different question types, due to their disciplinary training, whereas for other practitioners the need for knowledge about a sophisticated range of questions is less important. What we have presented here are five broad domains of question types that are all valuable and useful for different purposes in working with families that were recurrently evidenced in our own research data. We have illustrated that the use of questions is more nuanced than sometimes perceived and that it requires some skill to implement different question designs effectively. Thus, as a reflective practitioner, we encourage you to think about how you ask a question, why the design of those questions matter, and how different questions might work better in different ways for different reasons. As we progress through this chapter, we now focus on specific question types that perform various kinds of institutional business.

'Why Are You Here?' Questions

Ascertaining the child's beliefs regarding the reasons why they are attending the appointment with their family is important. Typically, the professional and parent/carer initiate and organise the appointment and thus the child is brought along to an appointment and may have variable levels of understanding about the nature, purpose, and goals of that appointment. A child-centred model of care prioritises inviting children to share their views and opinions about the process (Dogra, 2005).

> **Child-Centred Care**
> A practical implementation of a policy to respect children's rights to be involved in decisions that affect their lives.

Consequently, having ways to ask children about their perspectives is an important aspect of this process. In particular, ascertaining the child's understanding of the reason for their presence in the current interaction can be a valuable way to open the institutional task.

Although the institutional activity is considerably different across fields of practice, such as family therapy, family social work, mental health assessments, there is a universal value in consulting children about the reasons for their attendance. Our examples are drawn from our mental health assessment data, but nonetheless are translatable to any related context or setting.

Our data illustrated that the 'why are you here?' question was asked directly to the child in just over half of the 28 assessments, but in six cases the parent was asked instead and in two cases the practitioner offered up the reasons why the child was present at the appointment. In three assessments, the issue of why the child was present was not raised at all. Here, we report examples from the 17 cases whereby the question was asked to the child.

> Asking a closed 'do you know' question is likely to elicit a negative response.

There were three central ways in which children addressed this question. The first two were suggesting a possible diagnosis using mental health language or offering a vague description of difficulties or problems. However, the most common response was 'I don't know'. In the following three extracts, the enquiry to the child was formatted as a closed question. In each instance the child's response to being asked 'do you know why you are here?' was 'no'. Arguably, the child would have some concept for the reason for their presence, however the format of the question as closed, was not successful in eliciting useful responses.
(Taken from Stafford et al., 2016, p. 13, p. 14, p. 12)

Family 8 (Prac= Trainee Child Psychiatrist)

```
Prac    erm: (1.74) do ↑you (0.37) d- do you ↑know why ↑you're
        ↓here by the way?
        ((child shakes head))
Prac    no (.) not a not a cl↑ue
        ((child shakes head)) (1.04)
Prac    has mum not ↑told you ↓why
        ((child shakes head)) (1.13)
```

Family 16 (Prac = consultant child psychiatrist)

```
Prac     do you know why (0.39) you've come (0.75) to[↓day]?
Child                                                 [no  ]
Prac     you ↓don't (.) okay
```

Family 3 (Prac= Trainee Child Psychiatrist)

```
Prac     do you know> ↓why you are< why you- why you are ↓here?
Child    ((shakes head)) °No°
Prac     oh (0.59)
```

In this next example, the practitioner uses an open question to ask the child what their understanding is of the reason for the visit. However, the child still responded by stating that they did not know those reasons. Although the use of open questions is considered preferable to closed questions, our data demonstrates that children may have limited understanding of why they attend the clinical appointment (taken from Stafford et al., 2016, p. 10).

Family 6 (Prac= Consultant Child Psychiatrist)

```
Prac     why do you ↓think your: mum and ↓nana bought you
         here to↓day
Child    ↓don't know
Prac     don't ↓know (0.40) do you ↑think it's to ↓do with your
         behavio↓ur
Child    don't ↓know
Prac     don't ↓know ok do you think it's to ↑do with your
         ↑feelings
Child    ↓don't know
```

Despite the practitioner's effort to follow up on the initial question to the child about their understanding of the reasons for the visit, the child maintains that they do not know. Therefore, although question design is important, what can be learned from this is that it may also be important to take some time to explain the purpose of the appointment to the child before continuing with the institutional business. One of the valuable aspects of this part of the session is to build rapport with the child, to alleviate any anxiety they may be experiencing, and to lay out the goals and direction of the appointment. This is important as research has indicated that children tend to fear the unknown prior to engaging with services but do value being heard once they are engaged (Bone et al., 2014).

Using Why Questions

We highlight a specific form of wh-question here because these kinds of questions have created some tensions in clinical practice about the value of their use. Why questions are a specific form of wh-question that seek the reason or motivation behind something, and yet research shows that why questions are frequently heard as requiring an account (Pomerantz, 1980). In other words, why questions tend to be heard as slightly accusatory or implying possible fault. Thus, these kinds of questions can imply a challenging stance, such as blaming, criticising, or complaining (Bolden & Robinson, 2011). When working with children particularly, a why question may be heard as a challenge. It is therefore important to look at the function of a why question, the design of a why question and consider how these have been used in clinical practice with children and we turn our attention to this next.

In our own work on why questions in mental health assessments with children, we reported that there were three conversational contexts in which why questions were used (Kiyimba et al., 2017). First, was that the sequential positioning of the why question was important, as this question usually featured immediately after the child revealed something. Second, these could be indexically tied, in the sense that the practitioner could connect the why to what was said before it (e.g., why's that?). Third, typically why questions were framed in such a way which assumed that the child had the knowledge to answer, in the sense that the motivation or reason being sought was contextualised as something the child should or could be reasonably expected to know. We provide some examples of why questions being used in practice below (taken from Kiyimba et al., 2017, p. 231/2, p. 235).

Family 22

```
Child      No my cousin (only) told my dad (0.8) Ah:: my dad
           is stUpi:d
           (1.07)
           seriously
ClinPsy    ↑Why why d' you s[ay that?]
Child                     [he was riding b]ehind me yeah (.)
           when we're when me and my cousin was getting followed
           by the p'lice
```

Family 21

```
Adol*      I thought that she was gonna to come in and kill
           my family
CPN        Okay
           (1.3)
           Why would she do that?
Adol       >I don't know<
CPN        How old is she?
Adol       >Same age as me<
```

Looking closely at these two examples, it can be seen that the first one clearly elicits an elaborated response, whereas the second results in a claim to insufficient knowledge ('I don't know'). Ostensibly, there is a similarity between the two extracts, in that the why question follows a disclosure made by the child and appears to be a pursuit of further information. However, there are subtle differences that may relate to how successful they are in eliciting detail from the child. If we look carefully at the first extract, we can see that the child discloses a view of their father 'my dad is stupid …. Seriously'. So, the follow-up why question from the

> Bear in mind that a why question may feel accusatory to the recipient.

practitioner seeks to understand the reasons for the child holding a negative view of their father.

Importantly, the design of the why question is closely tied to the child's words and thus the practitioner's question closely aligns with the child's agenda. The question therefore facilitates the opportunity for the child to express more about their point of view. Notably, the second example is not as successful in eliciting elaboration. If we look at the alignment between what the child has said and what the practitioner asked, there is a slight divergence. The young person discloses a fear that his girlfriend 'was gonna [going to] come in and kill my family', rather than asking why he thinks that (or says that) like in our first example, the practitioner asks a circular question that requires the young person to comment on why he thinks she would want to do that. This requires the young person to imagine his girlfriend's motivation rather than explore his own reasons for feeling anxious. Thus, the practitioner does not maintain a close alignment with the young person's feelings.

In designing a why question therefore it seems important to consider that, first, they can be heard as accusatory, challenging, or requiring an account, and second, that it can be difficult to speculate about the reasons that motivate someone else's behaviour. Thus, our suggestion is that when using why questions it is most appropriate to keep the design and wording of the question tied to the child's thoughts and feelings and, if possible, use their own words. We offer some other ways of seeking reasons from children through question formats other than why in Box 4.1.

Box 4.1   Alternative Framings

Alternative framings of why questions
   Instead of asking a why question, other less direct formats for eliciting accounts include:

- What makes you say that? What makes you think that?
- What are the reasons for that?
- Tell me more about your thinking on that?
- How did you come to that conclusion?
- What do you mean by that?

> **Box 4.2 Reflective Activity on Using Why Questions**
> Reflective activity
>   Using why questions
>   When you are having conversations with clients, we encourage you to notice your use of why questions. Ask yourself—when, how, and for what purpose do you use why questions and how successful they are in acquiring accounts. If you record your work for supervision or other purposes, it may be interesting to relisten or look at a short transcript of your work.

We would encourage you to reflect on where a 'why' question might be useful for your clinical practice, and in what situations a 'why' question might feel challenging to a child or young person you are working with. Try the reflective activity in Box 4.2.

The Miracle Question

The miracle question is frequently used in many kinds of therapy to encourage clients to focus on how their lives may be different in the future in the absence of their current problem. Originally, the miracle question was devised as one of the four pillars of solution-focused brief therapy (De Shazer & Berg, 1997). According to de Shazer, the progenitor, the client's response is more important than the question itself (de Shazer, 2000). Thus, the collaboration between the practitioner and the client is a form of social construction, where moving forward in the dialogue is a negotiated accomplishment (Strong & Pyle, 2009). The miracle question has been widely used in mental health interactions. There are different ways of utilising the miracle question, such as:

- *If I were to wave a magic wand, what would you like to happen?*
- *If a miracle occurred in the night, what would that look like for you?*

- *Suppose tonight when you are sleeping, a miracle happened, what would that be?*
- *If I gave you three wishes, what would you wish for?*

> A well-placed miracle question can help set solution-focused goals with children.

It is accepted that the use of the miracle question in therapy is a helpful and solution-focused way of eliciting shared goals. However, our research has illustrated that if the child's understanding of the reason for attending the appointment, then children have a limited basis for contextualising why the question is being asked. Using conversation analysis to examine the sequences of interactions between mental health practitioners and children during mental health assessments, we explored one type of miracle question, which was 'the three wishes' (Kiyimba et al., 2018). This research demonstrated that when the child had presented their understanding of the presenting problem and accepted that they were experiencing difficulties with their mental health, they tended to orient to this in their first response (wish) to the three wishes question. A good example of this can be seen below (taken from Kiyimba et al., 2018, p. 423).

Family 1

```
Clin Psy:   ↑if you had three wishes (0.66) what
            ↓would you like to make happen
Adol:       ↑my OCD'd ↓go (0.38) away
Clin Psy:   °yeah
```

However, when the reasons for attendance had not been fully established and the nature of the presenting difficulties had not been fully explored, their initial response to three wishes was usually idiomatic and not related to mental health. Furthermore, in these instances, practitioners needed to do more discursive work with further lines of questioning to elicit goal-oriented responses. A good example of this can be seen below where the child's response of 'a million pounds' is contextually unrelated (taken from Kiyimba et al., 2018, p. 428).

Family 13

```
Registrar:       okay you've got three wishes what would
                 you wish to [see]
Child:                       [a million po]unds
Registrar:       [no (.) a million po]unds ok[ay]
Psychiatrist:    [ahh]                       [I ] would ↓like
                 th[at wish:]
Registrar:         [I'd love th]at as well
                 (0.38)
Registrar:       yeah o↑k (.) what else?
```

Arguably, mental health practitioners do not always establish with children what the reasons are for them attending the appointment (Stafford et al., 2016). While the three wishes question technique can be a useful strengths-based way to establish goals, it is important to first identify collaboratively what the problem is and therefore align goal setting with the institutional business. In other words, it is the sequential positioning of the question that is important for its success, rather than its specific wording. In this way, the miracle question is used in a way that relates to the institutional business. Another way to ensure the focus of the miracle question is to include reference to the problem in the question itself. The extract below, (from previously unpublished data) from our family therapy data, is a good example of this.

Clamp family

```
FT:        Now if if we if we could do some magic
Jordan:    Yeah
FT:        The three of y- the four u- if you Phillip you
           Ronald and you Jordan
Jordan:    Yeah
FT:        and me if we could be magicians .hhh and we could
           change things by magic (.) what would you change?
           (1.0)
FT:        what would you change Phillip? If we could get a
           magic wand .hh and we could wave this wand and
           cha<u>n</u>ge something in in your family (.) what would
           you ↓change?
Phil:      The <flapping> ((raises arms up and down))
FT:        Flapping (.) What's what's the flapp↑ing?
Father:    He flaps
Uncle:     He gets [so excited (.) when he's playing with cars
           or owt like that he'll sit there like ((flaps arms
           quickly))
```

The design of the initial miracle question is problematic in two ways, both of which relate to it non-specificity. First, non-specific speaker selection, as the therapist named all three children in the pre-announcement, and second, non-specific reference as the therapist referred to 'things' in general and change. Thus, following a 1 s pause where none of the children provide an answer, the therapist reformulates his miracle question in much more specific terms, first selecting Philip to answer it, and second specifying that the magic could change something about the family. This specificity is demonstrably more successful as Philip then provides a clear answer about what he would like to see changing, i.e., his flapping. This behaviour is relevant to his mental health and thus the institutional business of therapy, which is reported to accompany an emotion, that of excitement. We now turn your attention to the reflective activity in Box 4.3.

> **Box 4.3 Reflective Activity on the Miracle Question**
>
> Reflective activity
>   The miracle question
>   Now you have learned more about the value of a miracle question and the way to design a miracle question to encourage a child to focus on the goals of the session, we recommend you try this in your practice. Use a miracle question (if appropriate) in your next session with a family and after you finish, write your immediate thoughts in a reflective diary.
>
> - How was your question designed?
> - Did it work well?
> - Did the child engage?
> - Was the objective of using the miracle question achieved?
> - What might you do differently and why?

You Said Prefaced Questions

An awareness of the imbalance of power in the therapeutic relationship underpins the interaction, especially when working with children. The metaphor used in therapy to discuss power is that of resistance.

> **Resistance**
>
> Resistance refers to when the client does not cooperate with the therapist's suggestions, ideas, or questions.

Interventions are most effective when they "do not run counter to what the client desires" (de Shazer, 1988, p. 75). In other words, resistance can be avoided by maintaining a client-centred position that attends carefully to the themes, topics, and specific words of the client themselves. One effective way to preface therapy questions is to reintroduce the client's words using the phrase 'you said x'. The 'effectiveness' of the communication technique refers to; first, the eliciting of a response from the child, second, the response being relevant to the question asked, and third, that response containing some detail or elaboration. Through our analysis of the mental health assessment data, we identified that there were three core components to this sequence, which we outline in Table 4.1 (see Kiyimba & O'Reilly, 2018).

Table 4.1 The sequence

The sequence	
First part	'You said' question preface plus reflected speech
Second part	Recipient response slot
Third part	Question-answer

The first component following 'you said' was reflected speech which functioned as a preface to ask follow-up questions based on the reintroduced topic. We distinguish between reflected speech (Kiyimba & O'Reilly, 2018) and reported speech (Holt, 1996).

Reflected Speech

Reflected speech is typically 'you said' prefaced and used in the presence of the person whose words are being reported.

Reported Speech

Reported speech is typically 'he said/she said' prefaced and is used when a speaker refers to something that someone outside current action has said

The second component is the recipient response slot, which may include a verbal affirmative response from the client, or their silence is treated as implicit agreement. The third component consists of the practitioner's question and the client's response to that question; this is typically referred to as an adjacency pair (see Sacks, 1992). An example of this three-part sequence is provided below (taken from Kiyimba & O'Reilly, 2018, p. 152).

Family 1 (Prac = Community psychiatric nurse)

```
Prac     I'm ju↑st wo:↑ndering thou↓gh coz you (.) you said in
         the: (.) interview room that (.) it sta↑rted a couple
         of years ago [it FIRST]=
Child                 [yeah its]
Prac     = ever >st[arted] a couple of years ago<=
Child              [yeah]
Prac:    = so why↑ do you think it it started the↓n?
Child    January it could be sorting out changing thi:ngs (0.70)
         I th↓ink it could be like (.) say↑ing me (.) is coz
         like (.) I dunno (0.63) chan↑ging schools an
         th↓at li↓ke
```

This example illustrates the value of the 'you said x' prefaced question for eliciting detailed responses from the child. By positioning the discussion about the child's previous behaviour and when the 'obsessive behaviour' began, and in this way, child-centred practice is ensured. The effectiveness of this discursive technique is evident in the elaborated response from the child in the form of a disclosure of their understanding of when and why the behaviour started. This is particularly important for the practitioner to establish, especially in the context of a mental health assessment.

Circular Questions

Circular questions are frequently used in family therapy whereby family members are invited to consider the actions, thoughts, and feelings of other family members (Tomm, 1987a). Because of this, circular questions have also been referred to as other-perspective wh-questions (Lester et al., in press). It can be helpful for children to imagine the perspectives of others (Nelson et al., 1986) as this encourages their capability to mentalise. Mentalising is the 'ability to acquire knowledge about other peoples' beliefs and desires' and is thought to relate to the capacity to empathise with others (Frith & Frith, 2005, p. R644). Frith and Frith argued that the ability to mentalise allows the practitioner to assess the extent of the child's competency in theory of mind. Circular questions provide a mechanism for establishing and potentially challenging false beliefs. We provide two examples of this from our child mental health assessment project below (one of which we referred to earlier in this chapter).

Family 21 (taken from Kiyimba et al., 2017, p. 235)

```
Adol    I thought that she was gonna to come in and kill
        my family
CPN     Okay
        (1.3)
        Why would she do that?
Adol    >I don't know<
```

> Circular questions can be used to gently challenge false beliefs.

In the context of the young person disclosing a concern that his girlfriend was planning to cause him harm, the practitioner used a circular question to invite the young person's thoughts on what his girlfriend's intentions were 'why would she do that?'. The context for the use of this circular question indicates a gentle challenge of what might be an unrealistic belief that his girlfriend intends to kill his family. The young person's response 'I don't know' signifies that he does not have clear evidence immediately to substantiate his concern (and may also be a consequence of the question being 'why' prefaced—see earlier in the chapter).

Family 18 (previously unpublished data)

```
Child    (0.24) then walking back on my own (in it) and the
         people co- a bunch of people walk up to me (0.45) and
         start on me I'm obviously I'm gonna whip it
         ((screwdriver)) out and go if you don't (0.23) go
         away then I'm gonna use it (0.51) and just
         clear off so
Psych    S- so w what why do people ↓pick on you?
         (0.28)
Child    I I start it ↓most of the time
Psych    You start it
Child    Yeah but it's cus my I hang in the area
```

In this extract, the child is explaining his reasons for carrying a screwdriver when he is walking around his local area at night. He previously explained the need for a weapon for self-defence, and carrying a knife is interpreted by him as a risk of arrest and thus from his perspective it is reasonable to carry a screwdriver instead (contested by the practitioner). The child describes an example of a typical encounter whereby an unspecified 'bunch of people' walk up to him and 'start on me'. This is a colloquial expression for starting a fight (similarly, hang in the area is a colloquial expression for spending time in the area in a leisurely way). The psychiatrist appears unclear as to why people would start an unprovoked attack on the child and asks the circular question 'why do people pick on you?'. The question requires the child to mentalise about the thoughts, feelings, or beliefs of those unspecified others and to provide an account for their motives. In this case, the child provides an explanation by admitting that he is usually the one that starts the fight, indicating that it is not entirely unprovoked.

> Circular questions are useful for inviting a child's perception of other people's motives.

Final Thoughts

Questions are the cornerstone of communicating with children. Questions can open up or close down children's engagement with the institutional business at hand. Questions can reintroduce topics in a client-centred way, they can elicit multiple perspectives, they can encourage elaboration or reflection, they can seek information, and they can steer the agenda for the clinical task. Engaging children can be challenging and therefore practitioners need a suite of tools at their disposal. This chapter benefits from the experiential account of engaging children in practice from children's counsellor Michelle Youngs in Box 4.4.

Box 4.4 Practitioner Voice, Michelle Youngs

Practitioner voices
Michelle Youngs
School counsellor

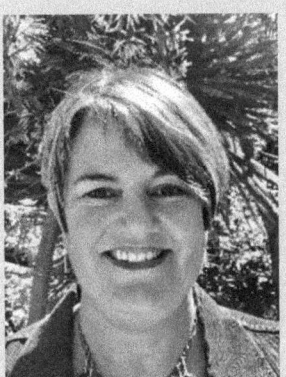

Michelle Youngs has a master's in narrative counselling and is an experienced school counsellor in New Zealand. Michelle is also an educator, training student counsellors in tertiary education.

In my experience counselling children, questions help to engage children, give the message to a child that they are significant and have something important to offer, invite a child to articulate their thoughts and feelings

(continued)

> **Box 4.4 (continued)**
> and give information to the therapist which helps inform assessment and direction. However, questions without a sense of rapport, connection, and playfulness are often experienced by a child as clinical or interrogatory. In many ways, the range of questions and depth of answers is correlated to the level of connection and trust the counsellor and child have. I tend to use questions in a playful way, particularly in the relationship-building phase. I use games such as Jenga which have questions written on them to get to know the child and for the child to get to know appropriate aspects of me. These reciprocal questions help to mitigate power giving more agency to the child. Questions around activities and subjects also increase a sense of child agency—for example, would you like to tell me yourself by drawing, the sand tray, the puppets, or talking?
>
> I find using a variety of types of questions effective depending on what is needed. A closed question to begin with often helps a child find their voice—"Hi, is your name Bertie?"—followed by more open-ended one—"I'm wondering what it was like thinking about coming and seeing me today…?" Miracle questions are magic once relationship is established and the focus is created. I find 'why' questions and 'when' questions often create confusion for young children—they often don't know 'why' something happened or 'when' exactly an event took place. I prefer to ask questions like 'I wonder what was in mum's mind when she suggested you come and meet me'?

In our experience of training practitioners, we have received feedback regarding the value of using naturally occurring data to explore using questions in situ to understand what works well and what does not. In this chapter, we have drawn upon some examples from our published works to provide practical methods for using questions in clinical practice. Some professions such as psychology, counselling, psychotherapy train in the use of different kinds of questions as part of their core training, but other professions may not have such depth of exposure. Thus, we hope that the practical tools offered here may provide some client-centred ways to ask effective questions of families and children. We summarise the key messages from the chapter in Box 4.5.

Box 4.5 Key Points
- Different types of questions are useful for different kinds of activity.
- Establishing the child's understanding of the institutional business can benefit engagement.
- Why questions need to be used cautiously because of their implicit account-seeking nature.
- Miracle questions work best when the child's understanding of the appointment agenda has been established.
- Using the 'you said x' preface is an excellent way to ask questions about previously introduced topics in a child-centred way.
- Circular questions are valuable for challenging false beliefs and inviting mentalisation.

References

Antaki, C., & O'Reilly, M. (2014). Either/or questions in psychiatric assessments: The effect of the seriousness and order of the alternatives. *Discourse Studies, 16*(3), 327–345.

Bilmes, J. (1988). The concept of preference in conversation analysis. *Language in Society, 17*(2), 161–181.

Bolden, G., & Robinson, J. (2011). Soliciting accounts with *why*-interrogatives in conversation. *Journal of Communication, 61*, 94–119.

Bone, C., O'Reilly, M., Karim, K., & Vostanis, P. (2014). "They're not witches…": Young children and their parents' perceptions and experiences of child and adolescent mental health services. *Child: Care, Health, and Development, 41*(3), 450–458.

de Shazer, S. (1988). *Clues: Investigating solutions in brief therapy*. New York: W. W. Norton.

de Shazer, S. (2000). *The miracle question*. Brief Family Therapy Center. Retrieved from http://www.netzwerk-ost.at/publikationen/pdf/miraclequestion.pdf

De Shazer, S., & Berg, I. (1997). 'What works?' Remarks on research aspects of solution-focused brief therapy. *Journal of Family Therapy, 19*(2), 121–124.

Dogra, N. (2005). What do children and young people want from mental health services? *Current Opinion in Psychiatry, 18*, 370–373.

Ehrlich, S., & Freed, A. (2010). The function of questions in institutional discourse: An introduction. In A. Freed & S. Ehrlich (Eds.), *"Why do you ask?":*

The function of questions in institutional discourse (pp. 3–19). Oxford University Press.

Frith, C., & Frith, U. (2005). Theory of mind. *Current Biology, 15*(17), R644–R645.

Hettema, J., Steele, J., & Miller, W. (2005). Motivational interviewing. *Annual Review of Clinical Psychology, 1*(1), 91–111.

Holt, E. (1996). Reporting on talk: The use of direct reported speech in conversation. *Research on Language and Social Interaction, 29*, 219–245.

James, I., Morse, R., & Howarth, A. (2010). The science and art of asking questions in cognitive therapy. *Behavioural and Cognitive Psychotherapy, 38*, 83–93.

Kiyimba, N., Karim, K., & O'Reilly, M. (2017). The use of why questions in child mental health assessments. *Research on Children and Social Interaction, 1*(2), 222–242.

Kiyimba, N., & O'Reilly, M. (2018). Reflecting on what 'you said' as a way of reintroducing difficult topics in child mental health assessments. *Child and Adolescent Mental Health, 23*(3), 148–154.

Kiyimba, N., O'Reilly, M., & Lester, J. (2018). Agenda setting with children using the three wishes technique. *Journal of Child Health Care, 22*(3), 419–432.

Lester, J., O'Reilly, M., Smoliak, O., Muntigl, P., & Tseliou, E. (2023). Soliciting children's views with circular questioning in child mental health assessments. *Clinical Child Psychology and Psychiatry, 28*(2), 554–566.

Nelson, T., Fleuridas, C., & Rosenthal, D. (1986). The evolution of circular questions: Training family therapists. *Journal of Marital and Family Therapy, 12*(2), 113–127.

O'Reilly, M., Karim, K., & Kiyimba, N. (2015). Question use in child mental health assessments and the challenges of listening to families. *British Journal of Psychiatry Open, 1*(2), 116–120.

O'Reilly, M., Muskett, T., Karim, K., & Lester, J. (2020). Parents' constructions of normality and pathology in child mental health assessments. *Sociology of Health and Illness, 42*(3), 544–564.

Pomerantz, A. (1980). Telling my side: "Limited access" as a "fishing" device. *Sociological Inquiry, 50*, 186–198.

Sacks, H. (1992). In G. Jefferson (Ed.), *Lectures on conversation* (Vol. I & II). Basil Blackwell.

Thompson, L., & McCabe, R. (2016). 'Good' communication in schizophrenia: A conversation analytic definition. In M. O'Reilly & J. N. Lester (Eds.), *The Palgrave handbook of adult mental health: Discourse and conversation studies* (pp. 394–418). Palgrave Macmillan.

Tomm, K. (1987a). Interventive interviewing: Part I. Strategizing as a fourth guideline for the therapist. *Family Process, 26*(1), 3–13.

Tomm, K. (1987b). Interventive interviewing: Part II. Reflexive questioning as a means to enable self-healing. *Family Process, 26*(2), 167–183.

Silverman, D. (1997). *Discourses of counselling: HIV counselling as social interaction*. Sage.

Stafford, V., Hutchby, I., Karim, K., & O'Reilly, M. (2016). "Why are you here?" Seeking children's accounts of their presentation to CAMHS. *Clinical Child Psychology and Psychiatry, 21*(1), 3–18.

Strong, T., & Pyle, N. (2009). Constructing a conversational "miracle": Examining the "miracle question" as it is used in therapeutic dialogue. *Journal of Constructivist Psychology, 22*(4), 328–353.

United Nations. (1989). *Conventions on the rights of the child*. UN.

5

Using Creative Activities with Children

Learning Objectives

- Be mindful of power differentials between practitioners and family members
- Identify ways to manage the power differential
- Use creative activities to support children in quantifying their emotions
- Appreciate the value of using symbols and archetypes to describe family systems
- Critically assess the rapid shift towards technological solutions

Introduction

The focus of this chapter is on engaging children and young people using creative activities. While there are therapeutic professions that specialise specifically in creative modalities such as art, play, music, or drama, our intention in our discussion here is more related to broader creative practices that can be utilised by any practitioner working with this age group. Referring to our datasets, we introduce creative techniques for accomplishing three of the common interventions that practitioners working with children and families are likely to find useful in their practice. From experience we have identified that these are: (a) finding ways to support children to express how they are feeling, (b) talking to children about managing anxiety, and (c) different approaches to gathering information about the child's family dynamics. We begin therefore by exploring creative approaches to talking with children about their feelings. The common numerical activity used with adults is the Subjective Units of Distress Scale.

Subjective Units of Distress

In a professional context, one of the organisational requirements might be to evaluate therapeutic outcomes, and both quantitative and qualitative measures may be used to collect these data. Typically, symptoms of anxiety and depression are measured pre- and post-intervention but may also be measured at each session or to evaluate efficacy. Other symptoms may also be measured depending on the presenting difficulties. A frequently used and simple rating scale is the Subjective Units of Distress Scale (SUDS). The SUD scale was developed by Joseph Wolpe (1969) and is used as a parsimonious tool to quickly assess a client's current feelings of discomfort (Matheson, 2014). This is a simple analogue scale typically represented from 1 to 10 measuring the subjective intensity of the currently experienced distress (Benjamin et al., 2010). These kinds of tools that examine emotions on a scale have also been referred to as scaling questions, such as in solution-focused therapies where scaling questions allow the therapist and client to jointly construct a way of talking about things that can be difficult to describe (Ratner, 2012).

Depending on the child's age, it may be appropriate to use a verbal scale of 1–10 to ascertain their state of affect. Notably, when using a verbal scale, it is important to explain that 10 represents the highest level of distress experienced and 1 is the lowest.

> It is important to keep both ends of the scale the same, i.e., that they both measure the same emotion. So, do not have happy and sad, have very happy and not at all happy.

The following extract is an example of this (taken from Kiyimba & O'Reilly, 2020, p. 420).

Family 3 (M=13 years)

```
Psychiatrist   Tell me about a scale of ten, ten being the most
               nervous, where do you rate yourself now?
Child          um five
```

However, for younger children, it may be too abstract to present the scale verbally, and therefore a more concrete visual representation is more suitable. An easily understandable metaphor for most children is to use a picture of some sort of vessel which can be constructed as empty or full or anywhere in between. In our data, practitioners used drawings of culturally recognisable vessels, such as jugs or teapots, to gather information about the 'level' of the child's current feelings of distress (Kiyimba & O'Reilly, 2020). Notably these metaphors were also used by practitioners to request information about levels of other emotions such as happiness or anger. The following extract is a good example of a practitioner showing a child a pre-drawn picture of a teapot and asking the child to point to the level on the teapot which best indicates how angry he is feeling (taken from Kiyimba & O'Reilly, 2020, p. 420).

Family 22 (M=11 years)

```
Clin-Psy    imagine this teapot is, we're gonna put all your
            angry feelings in here, yeah? how angry you'd get?
Child       yeah
Clin-Psy    if we were to take all the angry feelings out of
            you and pour 'em into this teapot how full
            would it be?
            (pause)
            you show me with your finger how full it would be?
            ((child indicates top of pot))
```

Although a drawing of a teapot was used in this example, there are many ways of undertaking this activity. Other vessels such as cups, bowls, vases, and glasses could be drawn, or it is possible to use real cup or bowl and ask the child to fill it up with water or sand. The advantage of using a physical object is that, depending on the therapeutic endeavour, some of the water or sand could be tipped out during the session as the child starts to feel better or to represent different time points related to an event. As an example, we provide a hypothetical script:

Practitioner: Using the jug of water and the bowl, think about how angry you were when your brother broke your scooter. Fill the bowl up to the level of how angry you were. An empty bowl means not angry at all, and a full bowl is as angry as you can possibly be.
Child: ((*Pours water into the bowl almost to the top*)). I was very very angry with him.
Practitioner: Let's imagine some of the things that help you to feel better when you feel very very angry. Let's make a list.
Child: I like playing with my dog Snoopy. I like riding on my bike. I feel better when I have a hug from my mum.
Practitioner: Okay, so, if you feel very very angry to the top of the bowl, and you have a hug from your mum, and play with Snoopy, does that make the anger in the bowl go up or down?
Child: It makes it go down.
Practitioner: Okay, so let's take some of the water out of the bowl.
Child: Yes ((*child uses the jug to take some water out of the bowl*)).
Practitioner: That's great. So, when you are at home and you start to feel angry you can remember to do one of those things that makes you feel better to bring down your level of anger, like we did today, scooping the water out of the bowl.

When working with children, it is important as a practitioner to be as aware as possible of the kinds of things they might be interested in, or play with, so that creative techniques can be used that are congruent with the child's personal experiences. In the UK, the use of a teapot as a vessel to creatively talk with children about the level of distress they are experiencing is culturally congruent because most households are familiar with the use of teapot. However, in another cultural context, this would not be a relatable metaphor and another vessel may be more familiar to the child. Younger children and those with developmental delay or neurological diversity may benefit from concrete use of objects rather than abstract concepts. For these children, it can be valuable to have a range of physical objects available such as containers that water or sand or beads (bearing in mind safe play and avoiding choking hazards) can be used to fill or empty. Another way that containers can be used as an intervention is when wanting to support children to identify ways to manage their emotions or stress levels is the stress bucket.

Stress Bucket

According to the stress vulnerability model we introduced you to in Chap. 2, the more adverse experiences a person has in their life, the more vulnerable they become to the negative impact of additional stressors. For children, the more adverse childhood events (ACEs) experienced, the more vulnerable they are to social, emotional, and mental health difficulties. One metaphor that can be used to talk with children about vulnerability and resilience is the 'stress bucket' (Kiyimba, 2020). The first factor to consider is the underlying vulnerability of a child that may be due to hereditary or biological factors. In the bucket metaphor, this would relate to the child having a smaller 'bucket' or capacity to manage stress than someone without those additional challenges. For example, a child born with foetal alcohol syndrome could be considered to have less capacity to cope with additional pressures in life. In other words, their starting point in life is to have a smaller resilience bucket than other children (represented in Fig. 5.1).

In the bucket metaphor, the next factor to consider is the number of adverse childhood events that the person has experienced. And this is represented in the analogy by the water or rain that is filling up the bucket. Another way of describing this is that every person has a finite capacity to cope with stressful events, and the more adverse events that person experiences the quicker they will reach their limit, as represented in Fig. 5.2.

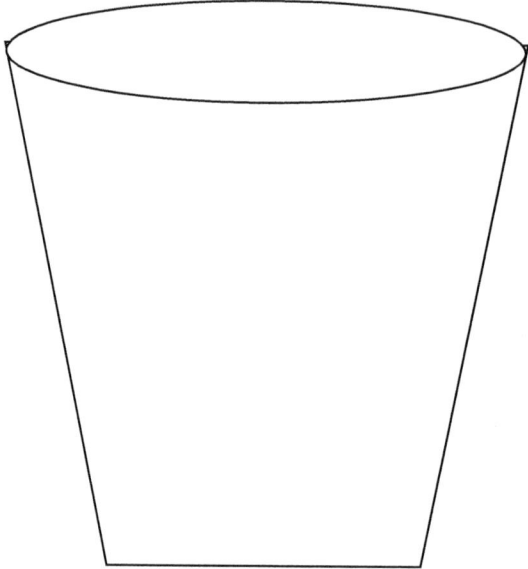

Fig. 5.1 Bucket sizes. (Illustrations taken from Kiyimba, 2020)

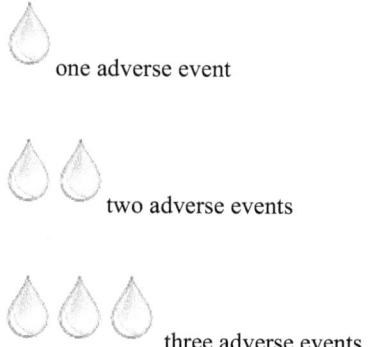

Fig. 5.2 Adverse events (taken from Kiyimba, 2020)

If a child has a smaller resilience capacity (bucket) to start with, and more adverse events (rain drops), the child's bucket will fill up quicker than a child with a larger capacity for resilience (bucket) and less adverse events (rain).

The value of this metaphor is to validate a child's levels of stress and distress and show visually how they might have a greater need to find ways to alleviate that stress than others. Stress relief can be taught by teaching coping strategies to enhance their resilience. In the stress bucket metaphor, the way this is described is by finding ways to either make holes in the bucket or to attach a tap so that some of the water can be drained away. The holes in the bucket or the tap represent coping strategies and protective factors that alleviate the pressure or harmful effects of the adverse experiences. This is represented in Fig. 5.3.

It is often not possible to reduce the number of adverse circumstances that a child is exposed to although this may be possible for some practitioners. So, it is often the case that the most practical support that can be offered to a child is to help them find ways to navigate the stressful events

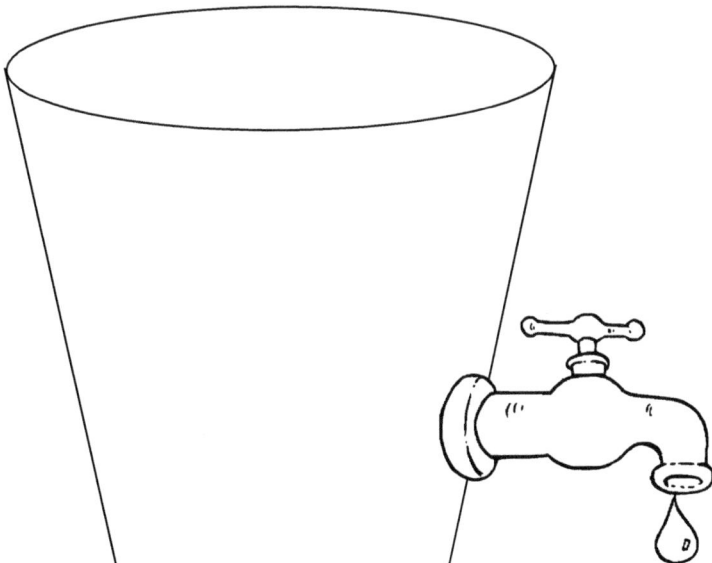

Fig. 5.3 Releasing the pressure

> **Box 5.1 Reflective Activity on Creative Techniques**
>
> Reflective activity
> Creative techniques—SUDS and buckets
> Imagine that in your resource box/cupboard in your place of work you have access to a range of plastic cups, funnels, and jugs. You also have paper straws and a sink in the room.
> We invite you to think about one of the children you work with and design an intervention using the equipment available that would be useful to facilitate a conversation about anxiety and stress management. You could draw on the ideas presented in this section or create your own.

and to incorporate coping strategies into their lives. For example, a small bucket with a closed tap might represent a child who has experienced several adverse childhood experiences (ACEs) or stressful events and has few coping strategies. In effect, their small bucket can be filled up very quickly with difficult life circumstances. To alleviate the likelihood of overflow, practitioners could support the child with ideas for stress relief and coping strategies that would in effect act as a way to open the outlet tap. The metaphor of the tap in the bucket can be used either as a pictorial illustration or with physical plastic buckets and water. With plastic buckets, it is possible to make a hole in it to bring the object lesson to life. Lists of strategies and protective factors can be elicited from children that would equate to ways in which they can help release the pressure from their lives.

In this section, we have introduced you to two related creative techniques for working with children in terms of measuring their levels of distress and finding ways to reduce that. We encourage you to engage with the activity in Box 5.1. to consider these creative strategies in your professional context.

Using Symbols and Archetypes

Symbolic representations are often used when working with families to map out and make sense of family connections and structures. These could be pre-existing symbolic maps such as those used in a family tree or could be created using readily available items such as buttons or shells. The idea is that the family members work together with the practitioner to collaboratively construct a two- or three-dimensional visual representation of their family system using the available creative resources. One of the advantages of creating a material representation of the family system on a piece of paper or whiteboard or table is that the family system and the relationships between family members are externalised. In narrative therapy, the use of externalisation of the problem is a key feature. The principle is that rather than the problem being located within specific individual(s), the problem is presented as outside so that the practitioner and client(s) can work together to find solutions to the problem (Tomm, 1989). Thus, potentially it becomes easier to have conversations about difficult relationships between family members using these external representations. One of the most widely recognised and used systems for representing relationships is the family tree. The following extract is an example of a practitioner introducing the family tree exercise to their clients (from previously unpublished data).

Clamp family

```
FT:        What I thought we could start by doing is to
           perhaps by drawing a family tree
Jordan:    Yeah
FT:        Yeah (.) Is that okay?
Jordan:    Yeah
FT:        Well, I'm gonna need help for this (.) because I
           don't know your family (.) and you know your family
           (.) yeah
Jordan:    Yeah
```

In this extract, the practitioner uses invitational language to offer the family tree exercise as a potential activity and solicits their agreement before proceeding. The practitioner uses the activity to position the children as experts in knowing about their family. Although this exercise is fairly simple, in this introducing this activity, the practitioner:

- Invites children into the conversation.
- Positions the children as experts in their own lives (equally this could position parents as experts too).
- Mediates the potential power differential between the practitioner and family members.
- Externalises the family system and in doing so externalises where the potential problem may lie. This is less threatening as it takes attention away from those in the room, onto the creative piece.
- Provides an opportunity for collaborative engagement between the practitioner and family members.

After introducing the activity, the practitioner moves to the next stage which is to navigate the technicalities of how to accomplish it. In some ways, this is presented as a game which has some simple rules, including squares to represent boys and men and circles to represent women and girls.

Clamp family continued (previously unpublished data)

FT:	I'll show you what we do to start with (1.0) what we do (.) I can't draw very well (1.0) I can't draw trees and things so what I do is (.) we're going to dra::w (.) a man (.) or a boy we put a square like that yeah so that's a man (1.0) or a ↑boy (2.0) and if we're going to dra::w (.) a:: woman (.)
Jordan:	Yeah
FT:	or a girl what sorts of shape do you think we could we draw for them? (3.0) What other shapes are there?
Jordan:	A circle?
FT:	And that's the right one yeah (.) we draw a circle (.) fo:::r a wo↑man (1.0) o:::r a (1.0) girl

In this scenario, the practitioner has been trained in how to do the family tree activity and in that sense is the expert introducing this exercise to the family. However, the way that they manage the potential power imbalance of taking an expert position is to mitigate that by using self-deprecating statements such as 'I can't draw very well'. Although in the family tree method, the standard symbols for male and female are squares and circles, respectively, the practitioner works collaboratively with the family by inviting their involvement in choosing the shapes. Similarly, the practitioner explains that in the family tree activity, a horizontal line between the shapes that represent 'two people' indicates being 'married' or living together as a couple and a vertical line represents any children they may have.

Clamp family continued (previously unpublished data)

```
FT         ↑now if two people live tog↑ether or if they're
           married (1.0) a man and a woman like that. what we
           do is draw a line between them (1.0) to show that
           they live together (.) and if they've got children
           we put a line down and we put the children down
           there like that (1.0) ↑yeah (.) shall we do that
           with your ↑family?
Jordan:    Yeah
```

After very briefly introducing what the symbols of circles, squares, and lines represent, the practitioner can move to language that includes more open questions and invites more ownership from the family about how family tree is created. In our example, the practitioner starts by asking who to 'start with'.

Clamp family continued (previously unpublished data)

```
FT:        Right (.) We'll leave that there so we can
           remember (.) the different (.) things (.) now who
           shall we start with? (.) What who shall we put
           in first?
Jordan:    ((raises his hand))
FT:        You want to start with yourself?
Jordan:    Yeah
FT:        Yeah, I think it might that's not a bad idea
           (.) but
Mum:       You can't ((shakes head))
```

```
FT:        I think we should start wi:::th (.) °shall we
           start with parents?°
Phil:      ((nods))
FT:        Yeah (.) with mums and dads (.) right so who shall
           we draw in first?
Jordan:    ((points to the father))
```

Ostensibly, the practitioner provides an open opportunity for the family to decide who the first person to be represented on the family tree is. However, the practitioner carefully guides the conversation so that the tree starts with the parents. In this kind of scenario when working with families, there is the risk at one extreme for the practitioner to dictate to the family how to go about the activity, and this may alienate them from the conversation. Additionally, this approach may detract from appreciation of the client as an expert in their own life (Anderson & Goolishian, 1992). At the other extreme, the practitioner might give too much control over the activity to the family members and lose the benefits of the structural knowledge that the practitioner has. Practitioners working from a social constructionist perspective would typically understand therapeutic collaboration as being fluid and dialectical rather than didactic (Larner, 1995). Practitioners working within a collaborative model would share their power with family members by "incorporating clients' meanings and preferences as part of their developing interactions" (Sutherland & Strong, 2011, p. 3). We represent the dialectical balance between the knowledge of the practitioner and the knowledge of the family in Fig. 5.4.

One way of describing this kind of 'both/and' positioning is referred to as the dialectic balance. This is a valuable skill for practitioners working with families to incorporate in their practice as it provides the

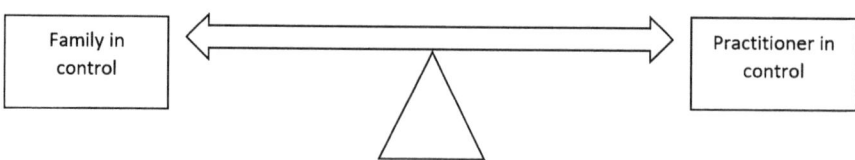

Fig. 5.4 The dialectical balance

opportunity to structure conversations with families in beneficial directions whilst also inviting the family to be involved collaboratively in the process. This process occurs in the continuation of the extract where the practitioner invites the family to decide what shape to draw to represent the father, and subsequently the mother. Although this is presented as an open question, the correct answer has previously been introduced by the practitioner as a square.

Clamp family continued (previously unpublished data)

```
FT:        Shall we put your dad in? and what shape shall we do
           for your dad (1.0) what shape?
Jordan:    E::r
FT:        Can you remem↑ber?
Phil:      Square
Jordan:    ((goes over to father and rubs his head)) Square (.)
FT:        That's right
Mum:       Heh heh heh
FT:        That one (.) what's that one?
Jordan:    Square
FT:        Square square so let's put your dad in there (1.0)
           like that and I always do these (.) too big (.) and
           there's not enough room
Dad:       heh heh heh
FT:        and there's not enough room to fit them in but we'll
           see how we go (.) and what shape are we gonna draw
           for your mum?
Jordan:    Circle
FT:        Circle (.) that's right
```

Once the basic 'rules of the activity' have been explained by the practitioner, there is opportunity to allow the family to have more ownership of how the family tree is collaboratively constructed in terms of the sequence of which children are represented first, second, or third.

Clamp family continued (previously unpublished data)

```
FT:      how many children?
Phil:    Three
FT:      Three (.) you're good at this you're getting (.)
         who's the eldest?
Phil:    Me
FT:      You are the eldest so we put you in first shall we put
         you in first? (.) Shall we put you in first?
Phil:    ((nods))
FT:      What shape are we going to draw for you?
Phil:    (3.0) Square
```

The previous series of extracts has illustrated one way that practitioners can work with families to co-construct a family tree. Family tree genograms have an established set of lines and symbols are used universally to represent the same characteristics in family systems. This can be useful for situations where practitioners might be working in multi-disciplinary teams and knowledge of this pre-existing system is helpful to share information between practitioners. Thus, this genogram activity has several benefits including:

- Provides information about the way that the family themselves construct their family system.
- Indicates losses such as relationship breakdowns, bereavements, and so forth.
- Illustrates blended family relationships.

Another way of working with families to create family systems maps is to use other easily available objects to represent family members. Some practitioners use buttons or shells or toy figurines to create family system models with their clients. Allowing family members to choose their own symbols can provide more opportunities for wider conversations about the characteristics of specific family members. This type of activity has several benefits:

- Potentially highlights areas of challenge in terms of relationships between family members.
- Provides a platform for idiosyncratic insights into how they see themselves, how they see other people, and the way that they see how people are connected to one another.
- Provides more spatial flexibility to place their symbol in a spatial location on the table or board in relation to their other family members.
- Allows a more kinetic involvement in a creative activity because family members chose and move around their symbol.
- Provides for a dynamic interaction where symbols can be moved closer to or further away from the symbols that represent other family members.

In reflecting on the benefits of genograms or symbolic activities, we encourage you to engage with the following reflective activity in Box 5.2.

> **Box 5.2 Reflective Activity on Using Symbols**
>
> Reflective activity
>   Using symbols in your work
>   In your professional and cultural context, consider what symbolic resources are available to be used with families to create family systems diagrams or models.
>   Consider how you might begin to incorporate the use of symbols in your family practice work or extend your use of symbols more creatively. We also encourage you to think about when these might be useful.

Notably in the previous section, we discussed the use of symbols which in their own right are neutral but can be anthropomorphised by family members to represent people. In the case of pre-determined symbols in the genogram system, this gives a structured way to gather the facts about family relationships. Using neutral objects three-dimensionally to produce family maps allows clients more flexibility to project their own subjective experiences and interpretations onto the object.

Another way to engage families in conversations about family dynamics is to provide archetypal images. Using archetypal images has the advantage of normalising certain 'types' of people by recognisable characteristics. For example, the characters in the fairy tale *Snow White and the Seven Dwarfs* represent recognisable archetypes, including 'the wicked stepmother', the 'handsome prince', and the 'innocent daughter', and each of the seven dwarves are also other familiar archetypes, such as 'grumpy', 'sleepy', and 'dopey'. Often family members will have an archetype from a culturally normative fairy tale, television programme, or film that they relate to, and discovering what this can provide valuable information about the way those members see themselves and what their core beliefs may be. In the following series of connected extracts of data, we illustrate how this type of activity can be useful in family practice (from previously unpublished data).

Niles family

```
FT:     Well, you don't have to think about yourself think
        about (.) people at school (.) when you see other
        children getting angry at school what do you think
        makes them angry?
Lee:    ((shrugs))
```

It appears that the practitioner in this extract is acknowledging that it might be difficult for the child to initially talk about their own feelings 'you don't have to think about yourself'. Instead, the practitioner suggests that the child thinks about other 'children at school' as a way to begin a conversation about emotions without it being focused directly on the child himself. The practitioner inquires what the child thinks might make 'other' children angry. Unfortunately, the child is still not able to engage with this approach and gives a non-verbal response of a shoulder shrug. The practitioner then takes a different strategy which further distances the child from talking about their own emotions directly by introducing the idea of working with archetypes. He does so by first inquiring about what television programmes the child enjoys.

Niles family continued (previously unpublished data)

```
FT:     What abo::ut on (.) what's your favourite (.) T.V
        programme?
Lee:    Simpsons
FT:     Simpsons (.) a::::h (.) what makes Homer angry?
        (1.0)
Dad:    D'oh
Lee:    His [son Bart
```

Using this strategy, the practitioner quickly establishes that *The Simpsons* is the child's favourite television programme. This refers to an animated comedy series about an American family and the antics that they get up to. Because the programme chosen is about a family, this lends itself well to the practitioner's agenda of finding another way to encourage the child to talk about his emotions in relation to his family context. Helpfully, the practitioner is familiar with the television programme and can name the father character 'Homer'. Additionally, because the practitioner is familiar with the archetypal features of the characters in this cartoon series, he can ask the question 'what makes Homer angry?'. This use of circular questioning to ascertain the child's awareness of someone else's cognitive reasoning is successful in eliciting a response that the cartoon character's son 'Bart' makes Homer angry. This resonates with the previously introduced dialectical balance figure, whereby the practitioner holds their own institutional responsibility in mind (to pursue a conversation about the child's behaviour), whilst also allowing the family the freedom to control certain aspects of how that conversation is shaped (by scaffolding the conversation around a familiar television programme).

Niles family continued (previously unpublished data)

```
FT:        Bart (.) what does Bart do that makes Homer angry?
           (1.0)
Steve:     Be naughty
```

As this short extract shows, the practitioner's strategy is successful in that the child answers the question about what makes the cartoon father angry, by replying it is the cartoon child's naughtiness that makes his father angry. While superficially the conversation still appears to be about *The Simpsons*, the therapeutic agenda is also implicitly moving forward towards a point where the practitioner can translate the archetypal family relationships in the cartoon to the current family dynamics. This is demonstrated in the remaining section of this extract.

Niles family continued (previously unpublished data)

```
FT:        So, if you were the Simpsons (1.0) … (.) if your
           family were the Simpsons (.) who would be Bart?
Nic:       ((Points to Steve))
Steve:     ((raises hand))
FT:        A::h
Dad:       heh heh heh heh
Nic:       I'd be Lisa
```

Having established a shared understanding about *The Simpsons*, the practitioner makes the transition towards a more therapeutic agenda by asking about the similarities between the cartoon characters and their family 'if your family were the Simpsons (.) who would be Bart?'. The humour and the collaborative production of the answer establishes the children's shared agreement that Steve the eldest child would be Bart, and his sister Nic would be Lisa. During the subsequent interaction, the practitioner collaborates with the family to draw up two lists, one of examples of Bart's 'naughty' behaviour and second list of exemplars of Bart's 'good' behaviour. Having completed the lists, the practitioner pulls the conversation back to alignment with the primary institutional agenda which is to focus back on the behaviour of the children in the room, but most specifically the child identified by the family as the one with the 'problem' (Steve). As demonstrated in the next extract, the therapist presents the two lists to Steve and asks him to write down the number of behaviours he and Bart have in common. Notably, the practitioner is careful to provide the child with some privacy by stating that no one else should see the list.

Niles family continued (following much more conversation) (previously unpublished data)

```
FT:    All you've got to do is look at these lists (.) I want
       you to write down on this bit of paper (.) >but don't
       let anybody see< all the numbers that are a bit like
       you (.) on the goo- on the naughty list and on the good
       list yeah (.) all the numbers (.) so if any of those
       are a bit like you you write the number down and then
       we're gonna ask everybody else to guess (1.0) which
       numbers you've written down so they're gonna guess
       which numbers you think are li[ke you
```

When the therapist asked Steve directly at the opening of the session what makes him angry and the behaviours exhibited when angry, the child did not provide a response. As a 14-year-old adolescent talking in front of his family, potentially his family are one of the reasons for the anger. The challenge of explaining himself when it may not have been talked about explicitly prior to the family therapy session could be too difficult for the young person to do directly. Therefore, this indirect approach was a more effective strategy, and the data illustrate that it is one that does engage him in the conversation. Although this creative approach using archetypal figures from a well-known television programme is a circuitous and lengthy process, it does have the advantage of providing a way for the family to be involved and for Steve in particular to recognise what makes him angry and how his behaviours might impact on others. For family therapists or other practitioners who want to take this one step further, using role play to act out alternative interactions can be a helpful creative approach to provide families with opportunities to experiment with different communication strategies.

A Shift to Digital

A digital revolution has transformed the way that people communicate across the globe. Most professions that work with families originated in a pre-digital era where face-to-face communication was standard. As such, professional training has in the past largely focused on developing skills in practitioners that support in-person interactions. However, the advent of a vast range of technological modalities has meant that most families utilise digital media, software, and technologies in their everyday lives. For the most part, practitioners working with families are still making a transition from purely face to face to hybrid working. In this section, we consider some of the advantages and disadvantages of the digital world and how practitioners can make best use of the opportunities presented. We focus on some of the ways that practitioners can engage in creative activities with families, mediated by digital health platforms.

Within the field of health, there has been a huge growth in the availability of mobile applications, with estimates of around 165,000 available apps in 2015 (Riaz, 2015). Some wearable apps, for example, can track sleep cycles, step counts, and heart rate. From a marketing point of view, these have been largely targeted at individuals for their own self-care, but some health practitioners may encourage their patients or clients to use these as an adjunct to their treatment plan. Within mental health, similarly there are apps that support people to be more mindful or to keep a record of their emotions and thoughts. Where previously practitioners might encourage clients to document this kind of information using pen and paper, the use of smart apps provides opportunities for recording, storing, and sharing that information digitally (Betton & Woollard, 2019). Furthermore, what is referred to as mHealth (for mobile devices) and eHealth (using electronic devices) has the advantage of global capability, meaning that people in majority world countries may also have improved access to healthcare through digital means (WHO, 2011).

Using computer-mediated communication has opened up new opportunities for the delivery of mental health care, especially since the repercussions of the global COVID-19 pandemic. Although there was some initial resistance to the necessity to deliver face-to-face interventions online, practitioners having had to transition to this modality began to discover the benefits of digitally mediated practice. Additionally, there were concerns that healthcare service providers required training in delivering services online as it raises different considerations including confidentiality, digital access and reliability, and visibility of physical cues such as body language. As such, Betton and Woollard (2019) argued that mental health practitioners require the appropriate digital skills and knowledge to deliver safe and effective care. In response, several regulatory or governing bodies of specific professions developed training resources for practitioners in transitioning their work to online. For example, in the UK, the British Association of Counselling and Psychotherapy (BACP) teamed up with the Open University which is an online education body to create a training programme for counsellors and psychotherapists to transition their work to an online environment. Apart from the informal opportunities that online support groups or bulletin boards afford, there are several different ways in which formal mental health care can be delivered. These can be asynchronous, such as email or text messages, or synchronous, through video conversations mediated by a web-based portal or instant messages (Mallen & Vogel, 2005).

The views of practitioners and families about the possible benefits of the digital shift have been mixed. For example, Cummings (2022) reported that practitioners working with young people's mental health found benefits in reaching populations that were previously difficult to engage. Similarly, Hoekstra (2020) argues that online treatment delivery can be valuable in reaching vulnerable families and have a lasting positive effect. Nonetheless, some cautions have been expressed regarding the challenges of managing safeguarding and privacy (Cummings, 2022). Parents and carers have also expressed benefits of digitally mediated therapeutic communication in mental healthcare, reporting a greater sense of inclusion through improved communication channels with clinical staff (Archard et al., 2022). Indeed, of the many research studies conducted during and after the COVID-19 lockdown periods enforced during 2020 and 2021, findings have indicated high levels of satisfaction with the use of telehealth platforms by both healthcare providers and recipients (Andrews et al., 2020).

Many people have come to recognise the benefits of using digital means as an alternative to face as an alternative to face-to-face healthcare, and researchers are confident that this is a promising viable way forward post pandemic (Andrews et al., 2020). However, for it to continue to be beneficial and sustainable, several legal, educational, infrastructure, and technical weaknesses in existing systems need to be resolved (Nittari et al., 2022). One of the areas that have grown in relation to the increased demand for digital health alternatives to face to face is the development of practice guidelines. Some of these are general, such as guidelines developed to consider environmental differences in the online space (Duane et al., 2022) or offer guidelines about training and service requirements (Thomas et al., 2022). Other guidelines are profession specific such as rheumatology (Ziade et al., 2022) or endocrinology (Vimalananda et al., 2022), and others are country specific (e.g., Australia: Toll et al., 2022) or ethnicity specific (e.g., non-Indigenous minorities: Truong et al., 2022).

Incorporating Creative Approaches Online

In this next section, we re-visit some of the creative approaches we have discussed in this chapter and provide some reflections on ways in which these face-to-face approaches might be adapted to online work with families. The first challenge to consider is that because families are not physically present in the practitioner's workspace the practitioner's tools, such as pens, paper, toys, and sand, are not available for creative activity. However, if families are in their home environment for the e-Health appointment they are likely to have access to other kinds of resources for use within the session. Therefore, it is possible for practitioners to invite families to gather paper and pens, or toys, or other creative tools in readiness for their appointment. For example, if we return to our section on SUDS, families could be invited to look in the kitchen for cups, jugs, or teapots, depending on what they have available. The practitioner could then talk them through the exercise while the child engages in a demonstration on screen as to how full or empty their emotion vessel is. Alternatively, it is possible to use the 'whiteboard' function on some videoconferencing software to draw images of a teapot or jug and invite the

> **Box 5.3 Reflective Activity on Creative Activities Online**
>
> Reflective activity
> Using creative activities
> We invite you to consider some of the families that you are currently working with taking into consideration your professional remit, your own technical skills, and the resources that might be available to those families.
>
> - What resources might families you work with have in their home that you could ask them to use during an e-health appointment.
> - How might using their own resources be advantageous or disadvantageous to achieving your professional goals?

child to colour it in, in a similar way to a physical piece of paper. We therefore encourage practitioners to consider ways to transfer creative activities into the online space rather than abandon them altogether. We invite you to engage in the following reflective activity in Box 5.3.

Some practitioners report that working online can improve initial engagement and can feel less confrontational to clients than face-to-face work (Furber et al., 2011). An interesting thing about working online with families who are in their home environment is that it can change the power dynamics of the practitioner–client interaction. For example, clients can choose to have their webcam on or off, although you may want to encourage them to have it turned on. Also, it is easier for clients to leave the appointment, if they choose to. Additionally, they may have more control over who attends the session and if creative resources from their home environment are used, they have more control over the choices they make about these resources. In some cases, it may be possible to record sessions and provide families with a recording which is less likely in face-to-face interactions. This gives families more control over watching the session again later and/or showing it to other family members at their discretion. We invite you to consider the diagram earlier in this chapter of the dialectic balance (see Fig. 5.4) and engage with the reflective activity in Box 5.4.

> **Box 5.4 Reflective Activity on the Dialectical Balance in Online Work**
>
> Reflective activity
>   Dialectical balance
>   We invite you again to consider some of the families that you currently work with or the possibility of working with a new family in your professional context.
>
> - How does the balance of power change between you and the family from in person to online?
> - What are the advantages of family members feeling more in control of the process in an online environment?

In addition to potentially having more control over the process, if the family are in their own home for an e-Health appointment, there is the possibility to use creative approaches to make the sessions more fun and engaging. If we return to the family tree example that we discussed earlier, in the face-to-face session, and consider how this activity might be approached in a virtual space there are several options including:

- Use the virtual whiteboard—and use names or shapes like on paper.
- Engage the children in photography tasks of acquiring images of family members to create a visual version of a tree on a digital cloud.
- Encourage the children to find items in the home that represent family members and talk about why they have chosen those items.
- Ask the children to paint or draw pictures of their family members that they can hold up to the camera or photograph and upload.
- Ask the children to make three-dimensional models with craft materials.

If families are on a limited budget and do not have access to resources, some practitioners are able to post out pens and papers to families in advance of the session. If resources are being posted out, an information leaflet for adult family members could also be included to outline what the session may involve. This leaflet may also include information or resources about further activities that could be done after the session.

Final Thoughts

In this chapter, we have provided a toolkit for practitioners working with children consisting of creative activities focused on talking about emotions, stress management, and family relationships. From experience we know that an area that children and young people often find difficult in professional settings is to talk about how they are feeling or to quantify those emotions. By providing suggestions about ways to support children via two- or three-dimensional creative techniques, we anticipate that readers will be able to use these skills and build on these suggestions with other ideas that fit the context and profession. The stress vulnerability model is an established and useful psychoeducational tool which we have translated into an object lesson that children could physically engage with to help them better understand the principles of stress management. In all work with families, an important part of our work as practitioners is to understand the family dynamics from the child's perspective. Using examples from our own datasets, we have provided real-life illustrations of how some practitioners work with family tree symbols and archetypes to help engage children in this process in a meaningful way. While our data and subsequent discussion provide a foundation for your own practices, these have been supplemented with reflective activities designed to support you to extend the suggestions provided in ways that might fit your professional context and client group. In Box 5.5, Sadiyya Haffejee describes some of her own creative practices in her work with children.

A foundational principle for practitioners working with children is to understand the world from the child's perspective. In doing so, the activities can be tailored to be appropriate for age, culture, and gender. Some of the techniques we have described in this chapter show how the practitioners in our data used open questions and an attitude of curiosity to find out what the child they are working with is interested in. The child's own reference point of interest may be a game they like to play, or a character on television they admire, or items in their environment they are familiar with. By identifying what is familiar and meaningful to the child, this can act as a starting point or foundation for the exercise that is professionally relevant. Most activities, such as the ones we described here

Box 5.5 Practitioner Voice, Sadiyya Haffejee

Practitioner voices
Sadiyya Haffejee
Psychologist

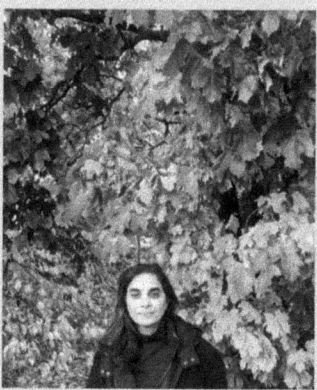

Dr Sadiyya Haffejee is a practising psychologist, researcher, and mum of two, living in sunny South Africa. Sadiyya works with young people that have been exposed to multiple adversities and aims to work in ways that are respectful. She draws on techniques that are compassionate and that foster connection.

Through my work in South Africa, I have been privileged to listen and engage with inspiring young people, many of whom have experienced significant adversity. Very often these children are unfamiliar with a therapeutic setting and may find it intimidating. Creative methods open up a space where children can express themselves in ways that feel less overwhelming and where they may have more control. Some of the techniques that have been most successful in my work have been mentioned in this chapter and include music and drawing. Other techniques I've used include the making of artefacts, such as mosaic treasure boxes and something as simple as walking and talking.

In using music, I may ask a young person to share their favourite song or a playlist they are listening to. We would spend time listening to a song and using the song to tap into feelings, memories, and key events. Inviting the child/young person to write a song has also been effective, especially when the child is very creative and already writing.

In drawing, I found that using timelines is useful in assisting children to recall events in their lives and structuring their thoughts. This also creates a

(continued)

> **Box 5.5** (continued)
>
> space where they can add both good and bad memories that are significant; and in this way recall the strengths and resources in their lives.
>
> A technique I find useful is the Tree of Life activity. This is a psychosocial support tool that draws on narrative therapy and was developed by Ncazelo Ncube and David Denborough (please see https://dulwichcentre.com.au/the-tree-of-life/). Using the tree as a metaphor, children are invited to draw a tree and imagine what it would be like to think of parts of their life as parts of a tree, with each part symbolising a different aspect. For example, the roots are where the child comes from, and the branches would represent the child's hopes. This process enables the telling of a richer, more nuanced narrative of the child's life. The focus on skills, and resources encourages a more hopeful story. This may be used before the child is engaged in the sharing of traumatic, challenging events.

> **Box 5.6 Key Points**
>
> - It can be helpful to track children's progress to use simple quantitative measures like the Subjective Units of Distress Scale.
> - It is important to maintain an attitude of curiosity and flexibility in how tools are used creatively with children.
> - It is helpful to think about the unique and specific aspects of the child in front of you when designing or using any creative techniques.
> - The starting point for imagining how to creatively adapt an intervention for a particular child is to find something of interest to that child.
> - Creative tools are a useful way of tapping into the multimodal ways in which children communicate.

including family dynamics discussions, can be conducted in numerous different ways and the principle of creativity in working with children is to combine the professional agenda with the child's agenda. We conclude this chapter with some final take-away messages in Box 5.6.

References

Anderson, H., & Goolishian, H. (1992). The client is the expert: A not-knowing approach to therapy. In S. McNamee & K. Gergen (Eds.), *Social construction and the therapeutic process*. Sage.

Andrews, E., Berghofer, K., Long, J., Prescott, A., & Caboral-Stevens, M. (2020). Satisfaction with the use of telehealth during COVID-19: An integrative review. *International Journal of Nursing Studies Advances, 2*, 100008.

Archard, P., Giles, I., Moore, S., Awhangansi, S., Fitzpatrick, L. K., & O'Reilly, M. (2022). Parent, carer and professional views of specialist child and adolescent mental health care during the COVID-19 pandemic. *Journal of Children's Services*.

Benjamin, C., O'Neil, K., Crawley, S., Beidas, R., Coles, M., & Kendall, P. (2010). Patterns and predictors of subjective units of distress in anxious youth. *Behavioural and Cognitive Psychotherapy, 38*(4), 497–504.

Betton, V., & Woollard, J. (2019). *Teen mental health in an online world: Supporting young people around their use of social media, apps gaming, texting and the rest*. JKP.

Cummings, A. (2022). The views of mental health professionals who use digital methods to support care-experienced young people. Social Work in Action.

Duane, J. N., Blanch-Hartigan, D., Sanders, J. J., Caponigro, E., Robicheaux, E., Bernard, B., et al. (2022). Environmental considerations for effective telehealth encounters: A narrative review and implications for best practice. *Telemedicine and e-Health, 28*(3), 309–316.

Furber, G., Crago, A., Meehan, K., Sheppard, T., Hooper, K., Abbot, D., Allison, S., & Skene, C. (2011). How adolescents use SMS (short message service) to micro-coordinate contact with youth mental health outreach services. *Journal of Adolescent Health, 48*, 113–115.

Hoekstra, P. (2020). Suicidality in children and adolescents: Lessons to be learned from the COVID-19 crisis. *European Child and Adolescent Psychiatry, 29*, 737–738.

Kiyimba, N. (2020). *Trauma-informed mindfulness: A Practitioner's guide for one-to-one work*. University of Chester.

Kiyimba, N., & O'Reilly, M. (2020). The clinical use of subjective units of distress scales (SUDs) in child mental health assessments: A thematic evaluation. *Journal of Mental Health, 29*(4), 418–423.

Larner, G. (1995). The real as illusion: Deconstructing power in family therapy. *Journal of Family Therapy, 17*, 191–217.

Mallen, M., & Vogel, D. (2005). Introduction to the major contribution: Counseling psychology and online counseling. *The Counselling Psychologist, 33*, 761–775.

Matheson, L. (2014). *Your faithful brain: Designed for so much more!* WestBow Press.

Nittari, G., Savva, D., Tomassoni, D., Tayebati, S. K., & Amenta, F. (2022). Telemedicine in the COVID-19 era: A narrative review based on current evidence. *International Journal of Environmental Research and Public Health, 19*(9), 5101.

Ratner, H. (2012). Introduction to 'Making Numbers Talk: Language in Therapy'. *InterAction, 4*(2), 48.

Riaz, S. (2015). Health Apps on the rise, but barriers remain, reveals study. *Mobile World Live*. From http://www.mobileworldlive.com/apps/news-apps/health-apps-on-the-rise-but-barriers-remain-reveals-study/

Sutherland, O., & Strong, T. (2011). Therapeutic collaboration: A conversation analysis of constructionist therapy. *Journal of Family Therapy, 33*(3), 256–278.

Thomas, E. E., Haydon, H. M., Mehrotra, A., Caffery, L. J., Snoswell, C. L., Banbury, A., & Smith, A. C. (2022). Building on the momentum: Sustaining telehealth beyond COVID-19. *Journal of Telemedicine and Telecare, 28*(4), 301–308.

Toll, K., Spark, L., Neo, B., Norman, R., Elliott, S., Wells, L., et al. (2022). Consumer preferences, experiences, and attitudes towards telehealth: Qualitative evidence from Australia. *PLoS One, 17*(8), e0273935.

Tomm, K. (1989). Externalizing the problem and internalizing personal agency. *Journal of Strategic and Systemic Therapies, 8*(1), 54–59.

Truong, M., Yeganeh, L., Cook, O., Crawford, K., Wong, P., & Allen, J. (2022). Using telehealth consultations for healthcare provision to patients from non-indigenous racial/ethnic minorities: A systematic review. *Journal of the American Medical Informatics Association, 29*(5), 970–982.

Vimalananda, V. G., Brito, J. P., Eiland, L. A., Lal, R. A., Maraka, S., McDonnell, M. E., et al. (2022). Appropriate use of telehealth visits in endocrinology: Policy perspective of the endocrine society. *The Journal of Clinical Endocrinology & Metabolism, 107*(11), 2953–2962.

Wolpe, J. (1969). *The practice of behavior therapy*. Pergamon Press.

World Health Organization. (2011). *mHealth: New horizons for health through mobile technologies*. WHO.

Ziade, N., Hmamouchi, I., El Kibbi, L., Daou, M., Abdulateef, N., Abutiban, F., et al. (2022). Telehealth in rheumatology: The 2021 Arab league of rheumatology best practice guidelines. *Rheumatology International, 42*(3), 379–390.

6

Children's Competence

> **Learning Objectives**
>
> - Recognise the ways adults treat children as competent or incompetent
> - Identify the ways in which practitioners can manage competency claims and assumptions
> - Critically assess the evidence on children's competence
> - Challenge traditional ways of thinking of competence as static

Introduction

The notion 'competence' has slightly different meanings within different fields of practice, such as psychology, education, sociology, and linguistics (Plaza Lara, 2016). The competence paradigm approach to mental health is considered an alternative to deficit-based models of practice (Masterpasqua, 1989). In relation to children, developmental theories are one of the main mechanisms through which the conceptual framework of children's development of competence has been perpetuated. Developmental theories propose a bio-cognitive maturational framework to suggest specific milestones through childhood. In building this understanding of children, neurodevelopmental perspectives added a caveat that some children may deviate from those standard norms. During their training, the study of developmental theories of childhood influences practitioners' expectations about children's normative abilities at different chronological ages. This has resulted in a view of children as 'incomplete versions of adults' (Danby, 2002, p. 25).

A more holistic perspective on child development and competency is therefore arguably needed, to account for the social, historical, and cultural situation within which the child is perceived (Burman, 2008). An alternative perspective on children's development and competency is that childhood and adolescence is a "*dynamic arena of social activity involving struggles for power, contested meanings and negotiated relationships*" (Hutchby & Moran-Ellis, 1998, p. 9). Thus, the traditional conceptualisation of a 'normal' child has been critically contested, with arguments presented that normality is created rather than revealed (Burman, 2008). For example, the neurodiversity movement advocates a different way of thinking about typicality and atypicality, which presents individuals previously positioned as 'abnormal' as a different kind of 'normal' (Ortega, 2009). In other words, competency is a socially constructed accomplishment that is co-created by iterative displays and uptakes within situated social interactions (Theobald, 2016).

In this chapter, we explore the idea of competence as an interactional accomplishment. The aim of this chapter is not to discuss the assessment of competency of children either formally or informally, but to explore the ways in which people treat children as being competent. One way of treating family members as being competent is to treat them as having access to certain areas of knowledge. For example, practitioners may display competence and be treated as having competence in relation to matters of the institutional agenda. Children may be treated as sufficiently competent to answer questions about their own thoughts, feelings, and motivations, but less so on more institutional matters. Parents and other adult family members are positioned typically as representing the 'middle-ground' having more knowledge of institutional matters than children and having more personal knowledge of their children than the practitioners. The domains of competence that we refer to throughout this chapter, as they relate to the datasets we include as example, and in terms of access to knowledge are:

1. Institutional systems, mental health, diagnostics.
2. Personal thoughts, feelings, mental states.
3. Competences to know or make inferences about the feelings, thoughts, motivations of others.

Situated Interactional Competence

Within institutional mental health settings, conversations are generally focused on the tasks of that organisational business and have distinctive features characteristic of the ways in which children express situated interactional competence (O'Reilly et al., 2019).

> **Situated Interactional Competence**
> Situated interactional competence refers to social capability to engage in appropriate conversational activities in particular contexts. In other words, the ability to converse with others conforming to conventional social interactional script within a specific situation or context (e.g., school classroom, doctor surgery, restaurant).

When we talk about social interactional competence, we do not refer to the clinical concept of mental health capacity. Instead, we refer to the social competence to be able to behave in an appropriate manner for the setting, and to articulate answers to questions in a way that is fitting to that specific institutional task. That is, we examine the in-situ competences of children by examining how their knowledge is displayed in particular institutional interactions (Bateman & Church, 2016). Thus, like Bateman and Church, we see knowledge as socially constructed, in the sense that knowledge is "constructed by and developed through interaction" (p. 5).

Rather than being a static trait or a single entity, we argue that children's competence is a dynamic accomplishment that may vary depending on the situational context the child is in. As such, displays of competence must be navigated in a range of institutional and mundane settings. In other words, the phrase 'displays of competence' speaks to the ways in which people behave to indicate competency in a particular area. For children, some of these settings may be completely new contexts that they have not encountered before and therefore the achievement of appropriate displays of competence is a social developmental matter.

One of the ways of developing social interactional competencies is to become familiar with the specific expectations or 'scripts' that are normatively established within certain environmental contexts. For example, there are normative scripts for behaviour in supermarkets, on the beach, at the dentist, in a café, in a school classroom. Clothing, behaviour, language, interactions with others, are all normatively modified in different ways depending on which of these social contexts a person is in. Edwards (1994, p. 211) described these kinds of scripted interactions as "typical or routine" and behaviour not conforming to those normative scripts would be treated as accountable. See the following examples:

- Wearing swimwear is normative at the beach or pool, but not in church.
- Singing is normative in a karaoke bar, but not in a library.
- Emoji use might be normative to communicate with friends in text, but not to your manager at work.
- It may be appropriate to run around in the park with siblings but would not be acceptable in the school classroom.

The characteristics of scripted interactions are that they are "recurring, predictable, sequential" (Edwards, 1995, p. 319). Arguably, almost every situated interaction has a normative script attached to it that has these characteristics.

The term 'deontic reasoning' is used to refer to the ability to understand and recognise the social rules of different social situations (Schaarschmidt, 2018). Usually, individuals from a shared cultural background would assume a shared scripted knowledge of familiar events, venues, and institutions. For the most part, unless these social norms are transgressed, people do not need to explain schematic expectations to each other, or even give them much thought, because of this shared deontic basis. Therefore, because of culturally shared epistemic and deontic understandings of social situations, people tend to only explain a normative script to someone else when they anticipate the other person may be unfamiliar with that script. For example, for a child who has never visited a dentist, a parent might explain before they go what to expect. Similarly, an older relative who has not previously visited an internet café before may need some guidance on what to expect. As people encounter different situations and contexts during their life, they become more familiar with a wider range of different event- and situation-specific scripts. The development of these scripts is culturally determined as different countries have different norms for events such as weddings or funerals, and different conventions for behaviour during meals.

A child's familiarity with specific context-related scripts will be determined by their age and the number of opportunities they have had to observe or engage in that activity or encounter that setting. In relation to mental health settings, some children may have had numerous encounters with mental health practitioners in early childhood and might have familiarity with the kinds of scripts to be anticipated. However, for some children, experience of these settings will be completely new, and they have not yet developed a frame of reference to know what might be expected of them. This lack of knowledge about the setting and expectations can lead to some anxiety for children when attending mental health services for the first time (Bone et al., 2014). For example, in the following extracts taken from an interview study with children who had recently attended Child and Adolescent Mental Health Services (CAMHS) for the first time, the data illustrate that the lack of prior knowledge of what to expect was anxiety provoking (taken from Bone et al., 2014, p. 452).

> Respondent: I was a bit scared.
> Interviewer: You were a bit scared? Can you remember what you felt a bit scared about?
> Respondent: I didn't know what we were going to do.
> (Child 9)

In the following extract, the interviewer asked the child what advice they would have for other children who might need to access CAMHS for the first time and might be worried about it (see Bone et al., 2014, p. 453).

> Interviewer: . . . if he was feeling worried about going to see CAMHS, what do you think?
> Respondent: Just don't because they're not witches . . .Just say that it'll help you out.
> (Child 8)

In the absence of knowing what to expect the child had created a concern in his mind about the practitioners being 'witches' and discovered only through experience that this was unfounded. This is a good example of situated interactional competence not being a static internal trait of a child but one that is dynamic and experientially developed. Generally, institutional contexts are less frequently encountered in a child's life, than mundane settings like the home or park. An exception to this is the school setting which is arguably the main reference point for a child's understanding of the general category of institutional script.

The difference between mundane and institutional-scripted situations lies predominantly in the formality or informality of those settings. Formal institutional settings tend to have similar parameters on behaviour which compared to mundane settings are generally more restricted. In other words, institutional settings place certain constraints on behaviour and to be able to display social competence an awareness and adherence to these constraints is required (Hutchby & Moran-Ellis, 1998). For example, in a school classroom environment children would typically be expected to sit at desks and be quiet while the teacher is speaking and constrain their urges to act otherwise. Similarly, in the institutional settings where most mental health practitioners engage with families, there are similar expected constraints on children's behaviour. When there are parents present in a family session, they can take responsibility to ensure that children behave in an appropriate way for the context. However, when children are seen on their own, especially for the first time, the onus is on the practitioner to provide guidance to the children as to what the expectations are for that interaction.

Previous research has indicated that children frequently claim lack of knowledge about the reasons for their attendance at a mental health clinic, typically using the phrase 'I don't know' in response to questions about the purpose of the appointment (Stafford et al., 2016). The value of providing children with more information about what to expect in an unfamiliar institutional context is several-fold; from an ethical point of view, children should be provided with enough information to give their consent; and from the point of view of minimising anxiety about the unknown, the effectiveness of the interaction will be increased if the child is calmer. Our recommendation from the evidence base, therefore, is that it is helpful for mental health practitioners to articulate what the 'script' of a first visit might be and what a child or family might expect. Similarly in the first session, it can be helpful for practitioners to outline what the structure of the session might be and what the practitioner plans to do, and how they plan to involve different family members.

> The onus for explaining an institutional script to a family is on the mental health practitioner.

The following extract is a good example of how this can be managed in practice (previously unpublished data). The psychiatrist begins the session by taking time to explain to the child what to expect and gives the child permission to ask questions if she is unsure.

Family 6

```
Psych     ↓k ↑what's gonna happen tod↓ay is we are going to ↓ask
          (0.78) probably your m↓um and your ↓nana some
          ↓questions and you as ↓well (0.30) yeah
          (0.23)
          we're gonna start off to↓gether but then what we are
          going to ↓do is I'm going to probably see you ↓on your
          ↓own to do some (0.40) drawing and some ↓games with
          you to just find out how things are from your point of
          ↓view (0.28) whilst (name) ↓speaks to yo:ur (0.24) mum
          and ↓nana (0.44) yeah
          (0.61) ((child nods head))
((Lines omitted))
          its ↑very important that if ↓you're not sure about
          ↓what's going o:n (0.30) or you don't underst↓and
          something that you kind of ask ↓us cause ↓this is
          about (.) you
          (1.07) ((child nods head))
          o↑kay (0.43) so its really imp↓ortant that you kind of
          ↓know (0.38) what we're ↓talking about and why we're
          ↓talking about (0.84) that (1.04) ↑okay
          (1.70)
          any questions be↓fore I carry on?
          (0.51)
          ↓is that ↑all reasonably ↑clear?
          (0.46) ((child nods head))
```

Although your professional context is very familiar to you in terms of expected normative behaviour, clothing, language, and so forth, these normative scripts may be completely unfamiliar to families, especially if they are engaging with services for the first time. We therefore encourage you to engage with the activity in Box 6.1.

> **Box 6.1   Reflective Activity on Preparations**
>
> Reflective activity
>   Preparations
>   We invite you to reflect on an unfamiliar place you have been to or an unfamiliar event that you have attended. Reflect on how you felt. Consider what preparations you made to try to predict what would be socially appropriate in terms of clothing and behaviour in that context.
>   Consider the clients you work with and how they might be feeling on their first encounter with you in your professional context. What steps could you take to support and prepare those family members to know what to expect.

The Knowledge Continuum

Depending on whether a person has engaged in a specific institutional context previously, they can be expected to have more or less knowledge of what the script for that type of interaction might be. To explore this further, we draw upon a theoretical approach that utilises the framework of a continuum along which some members of the interaction may have more knowledge (K+) and other members of the interaction may have less knowledge (K-) in different domains (Heritage, 2012). Some scholars refer to this as an epistemic gradient (Heritage, 2012), but within a practice-based context, the notion of a knowledge continuum is more congruent with the family interaction discourses associated with mental health.

In mental health settings, practitioners are typically positioned by self and others as being closer to the K+ end of the continuum, with parents and adult family members being closer to the centre, and children being closer to the K- end. See Fig. 6.1.

In an institutional context, the individuals with the greatest knowledge (K+) of the institutional agenda, script, and vocabulary, are the mental health practitioners. In this context, the individuals with the least knowledge (K-) of institutional expectations are the children of families in

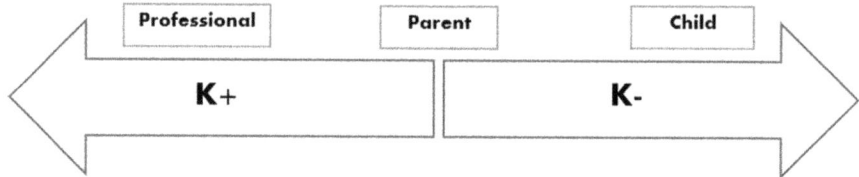

Fig. 6.1 K+-K- knowledge continuum in relation to institutional knowledge

attendance. Positioned mid-way between these two extremities of K+ and K- are adult family members who are likely to have some knowledge of institutional scripts, but not as much as the practitioners, and some knowledge of their child, but not as much as the child themselves. Thus, they occupy the mid-point on the K+ K- continuum by virtue of being non-practitioner adults. In general, the literature describes children as having less knowledge in most contexts than adults.

Another way of describing children as having less knowledge or being in a K- position is that in a conversation that includes adults, children can be treated as only having 'half-membership' (see Hutchby & O'Reilly, 2010). Thus, we recognise that agency, causality, and power are neither static nor unilateral in conversations between adults and children (see Kuczynski, 2003). Yet, there is some literature that illustrates that in healthcare interactions, children are more likely to be treated as not being full interactional members of the conversation and are not afforded the same rights to speak or contribute in the same way as adult members (O'Reilly, 2008; Stivers, 2001, 2012). Although when practitioners take steps to manage the adult-controlled interactions and support the child, children can manage to solicit parental assistance in answering questions without losing the chance to present their own accounts (Clemente, 2009). The disparity between adult- and child-perceived competencies in the unfamiliar institutional context of a mental health setting, is arguably further exacerbated by children having less familiarity with the script expected in that environment. In addition, it is often the case that the child may have a mental health difficulty that further impacts on their capacity to display interactional competence in these settings (O'Reilly et al., 2019).

Institutionally Situated Linguistic Competence

In relation to children's developmental competence in learning about the various interactional scripts that are normatively expected in different settings, we have previously examined children's behaviour and relative status in adult-child conversations. In this section of the chapter, we consider children's linguistic competence as it relates to the expected language scripts of institutional mental health contexts. The language of mental health practitioners is typically oriented to diagnostic terminology and the relationships between these diagnostic categories and symptom clusters. Thus, mundane ways of describing physical sensations, emotions, thoughts, and behaviours are transformed by mental health practitioners into a very specific range of linguistic terms. Words like 'disorder', 'condition', and 'illness' are the realm of the mental health practitioner. Potentially, then, there is a possible disparity between the linguistic repertoire of the mental health practitioner and the family members with whom they are interacting. Evidence suggests that family members, including children, attempt to bridge this gap by utilising medical or pseudo-medical terminology to describe their experiences. The following extract is an example of a child trying to engage with the institutional discourse of medicine (taken from Stafford et al., 2016, p. 8/9).

Family one (Prac = clinical psychologist)

```
Prac     ↑Do you kno:w (0.31) why you've c↑ome here toda↓y?
Child    erm because (0.39) I- keep (0.94) doin my- (0.41) I
         thi↑nk it's ↓O- C- D-
```

In response to the practitioner's question to the child about reasons for attendance, the child seems to frame the start of their answer in a mundane linguistic framing *'I keep doin' my'*. However, the child quickly repairs this mundane formulation to utilise a more institutional linguistic framing *'I think it's OCD'*. This demonstrates the child's orientation to the institutional setting and therefore a display of linguistic competence. The response from the practitioner questions this level of linguistic competency, as can be seen in the next part of the extract.

Continued...

```
Prac     Ri:ght (0.78) ↑ok:(0.92)um (0.52) °that is a (.)
         important word you use° (.) m↑eaning when you say O- C- D-
Child    °pard[on-]°
Prac          [ah ] wh- when you say O- C- D- what does it me:an?
Mum      whad'ya think it me:ans when you say O- C- D-
Child    um-(1.10) Ah: can't remember what the teacher to↑ld me-
```

Although the child utilises an appropriate medical terminology for the setting, and potentially the correct diagnostic label, the practitioner displays caution and seeks clarification from the child about what he/she understands that term to mean. In this way, the practitioner has not immediately accepted the child's offered candidate diagnosis, but rather has sought to establish greater meaning in terms of the behaviours or symptoms that might have led to that understanding. In other words, practitioner required more information to accept the assertion made by the child to explore how accurate that medical term may be. Evident from the practitioner's questioning, is that the behaviours of the child are within the child's epistemic domain to be reported, yet the medical terminology is not necessarily treated as within the child's epistemic domain, and thus requires further attention. Thus, regarding competency, children are not treated as either having competence or not, but rather competency is a more subtle and sophisticated interactional accomplishment. Children may be treated as having expected competency in one area, and not expected to have competency in another.

Competence to Report One's Own Motivations, Feelings and Thoughts

In relation to the epistemic continuum, in an institutional setting, the practitioner is assumed to have more institutional knowledge (K+) than the family members, including knowledge of specialist areas, like health,

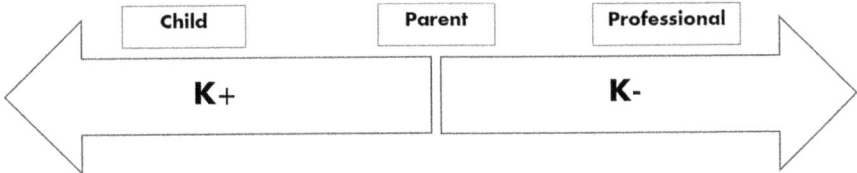

Fig. 6.2 The knowledge continuum reversed

social work, and education. However, it is frequently the case that family members and children are treated as having personal knowledge of aspects of their own life, including personal experiences such as their own thoughts, intentions, and emotions. In relation to the domain of institutional business, the family members may be in a K− position, but in terms of the domain of personal knowledge, they are K+ position. See Fig. 6.2.

Thus, in relation to the knowledge continuum, children are typically not expected to have very well-developed knowledge of institutional systems but depending on their developmental age and capacity for psychological insight they are expected to be able to access and report on mental and emotional states. Therefore, they occupy the K+ position (see figure), whereas the practitioner will occupy the K− position (see figure). Once again, adult family members retain a mid-way position having some knowledge of their child's internal states by virtue of close familial proximity and having spent a lot more time with the child than the practitioner.

The way that this can be seen in family interactions with practitioners is that the practitioner will display an assumed level of competency in the child and treat them in the design of their question as having the competence to answer questions about their inner states appropriately. In other words, the child is treated as being in a K+ position in relation to self-knowledge. In his original lectures pioneering conversation analyst, Harvey Sacks (1992) noted that people display expectations of interactional competency in their conversational turn-taking. He argued that recipients are treated as having unique access to their own inner states and of being capable of articulating what those things are. Similarly, in the data that we present, practitioners treated children as having interactional competence to appropriately respond to questions about their inner states.

In working with children in family mental health interactions, practitioners tend to recognise that the emotional literacy of some children will relate to their family circumstances and developmental stage. Indeed, the focus of the work of the practitioner may be to help them identify emotions they are feeling and learn to articulate those feelings verbally rather than behaviourally. In phrasing questions about experiences, thoughts, and feelings, while there is a general assumption of competency, in the mental health context, this may be an area of exploration with family members. Nonetheless, starting from the place of competency and if the child struggles, then this K+ and K- continuum can be used as a positive tool for intervention. In other words, asking children questions from a K+ oriented position initially provides the opportunity for them to contribute a K+ or K- answer. However, if a practitioner assumes the child is in a K- position initially, it is unlikely the questions the practitioners ask will give the child the opportunity to say things they want to (thus, they are assuming the child will not be able to answer that question). We provide examples of both situations.

The following extract is an example of the practitioner demonstrating anticipated K+ competency when he asks the child questions about his thoughts and feelings (taken from O'Reilly et al., 2016, p. 907). In the second part, the child's response demonstrates situated interactional competency by responding in an institutionally appropriate way.

Family 21

```
Prac      What do you THINK will happen if you don't touch
          something that's light?=
Child     = The worry in my head will come real.
Prac      The worry in your head [will c]ome ↓real
Child                            [yeah]
Prac      (0.2) What's the worry in your head?
Child     Could be anythink
          (.)
Prac      Give me the a a an example of one of the worries that
          you might have
          (0.2)
Child     Somebody will die.
```

In his/her initial turn, the practitioner demonstrates an expectation of K+ when they ask the child about their thoughts. The child demonstrates K+ competency in response by explaining what their worry is. This is further explored by the practitioner when they ask specifically for an example. Again, the child can demonstrate competency within the domain of K+ about their own thoughts and feelings. The following extract is an example of an instance where the child is treated as being in a K+ position about a personal experience, but the child articulates a response that claims a K- position on that subject (taken from O'Reilly et al., 2016, p. 907).

Family 2

```
Prac     and I ↑wonder if you ↓could (0.5) ↑just tell me about
         ↑how things were ↓when you were (.) small ↓whether you
         went to (0.8) nurse↑ry pl↓ay gr<u>ou</u>p?
Child    ((shrugs shoulders)) ↓Can't remem[ber heh heh] heh
Prac                                      [(No) heh heh]
```

The practitioner in this extract indicates an expectation that the child will have K+ knowledge about attending a nursery or play group when they were younger. However, the child claims a K- position by reporting that he/she *can't remember,* thus refuting the assumed K+ position on that topic. The laughter that constitutes part of the child's K- turn, also perhaps displays some discomfort in articulating that epistemic position, which may reflect a sense of accountability. In other words, when the practitioner positions the child as having anticipated K+, in doing so they display an expectation that the child would know the answer. However, the child may experience this as an expectation that they should know. Thus, there is a delicate balance between treating a child with competency, but not making them feel too uncomfortably accountable if they take up a K- position.

Knowledge of the Feelings and Thoughts of Others

So far, we have used the K+ K- continuum model to illustrate the ways in which practitioners, adult family members, and children occupy different knowledge positions depending on the domain of knowledge under discussion. However, a slightly more complex area of potential knowledge and competency to report on is the area of other people's thoughts, feelings, and motivations. We invite you to reflect on this more challenging domain of knowledge and competency by addressing the activity in Box 6.2.

So far, we have shown that practitioners generally treat children as having unique access to their own thoughts and feelings and the examples presented previously illustrated how this was demonstrated in practice. However, in mental health settings, it is common for practitioners to ask children to think about the thoughts, feelings, and motivations of others, often other family members. One of the reasons for this, therapeutically, is to assist the child in considering the possible impact of their behaviour on other people; in other words, to imagine what others may be thinking or feeling. When a child is able to articulate an understanding of mental states, it is referred to as a theory of mind (Sodian et al., 2020). To ascertain this, a practitioner might ask a child *'how does mum feel about that?'* or *'what do you think your brother might think if you did that?'*. These kinds of circular questions help children develop their theory of mind (Wellman, 1990) and empathy for others. However, from a K+ K− perspective,

---

Box 6.2 Reflective Activity on Access to Knowledge of Other People

Reflective activity
  Knowledge continuum
  Using the K+ K− continuum, consider where you would position these three hypothetical characters to be able to answer the following questions asked to the child's mother.

- "What do you think the GP might think about your child's behaviour?"
- "How do you feel about your child's behaviour?"
- "Why did your child throw their bag across the floor?"

For each question, who do you imagine would be in the K+ position, who would be in the K− position, and who would be in the middle, to answer these questions? (The GP, the mother, or the child?)

We suggest you draw a figure (like the one we have provided earlier) to illustrate your choice of positionings in relation to who would have the most competency to occupy a K+ position, and who might be expected to have the least knowledge.

knowledge about other people's internal states can only be inferred from how they behave and what they say and is therefore more difficult to assess. In terms of interactional competency, being able to articulate what someone else might be thinking or feeling is a greater epistemic challenge for the child. The following data extracts are examples of family members being asked questions about other family members' mental states (previously unpublished data).

Family 27

```
CPN        °°Okay.°° So- so mum's just looking at other schools.
           .hhh Wh::y (.) why d'ya think mum's looking at other
           schools?
Child      Prob'ly ter:::  find .hh children like me.
           (1.0)
           So a:h can:: <intr'act> wi'↑them
CPN        °Okha:y.°
```

Oak clinic

```
Therapist: D'you think he still sees himself as naughty?
           (3.0)
Mother:    I ↑don't know, I think he can now identify (0.7)
           that he has done, in certain areas he has done
           things wrong
```

In both examples presented, the practitioners ask the family member what they *'think'* might be the internal state of another family member. In the first example, the practitioner asks the child to speculate about the reasons why their mother is seeking to identify an alternative school. In the second example, the practitioner asks the mother to offer her perspective of her son's perception of himself as *'naughty'*. Asking what the recipient thinks, provides the opportunity for a range of potential responses (in contrast to asking what they know, which would presuppose a correct answer). In this way, the design of the question allows for the question recipient to provide their own perspective. In both examples, in response to this kind of question formulation, the recipient provides an appropriate response. In the following examples, the practitioner's question does not include the *'why do you think'* component, and illustrate that recipients have more trouble in answering questions formulated in this more direct way (from previously unpublished data).

Family 21

```
Child    I don't know why= I keep thinking ↓someone's standin'
         be'ind me now (0.6) don' know if it's the cameras or
         anyfink (0.7) I always get that when I'm walking keep
         thinking someone's (.) following me
CPN      why would they do that to you?
         (1.2)
         why would somebody want to follow you?
Child    I don't know
```

In response to the practitioner's initial question about the motivations of the person described by the child *'why would they'*, the child does not respond and instead there is 1.2 s silence. Again, when the practitioner asks a further question about *'why would somebody'* the child is unable to answer and states *'I don't know'*. The fact that the questions which do not include the caveat *'why do you think'* are not answered by the recipient suggests that this question formulation is more difficult to answer. This is because the inclusion of an invitation to state what they 'think' allows the respondent to speculate and explore a range of possible answers, rather than state definitively an implied 'correct' answer.

> Asking questions that begin *'why do you think'* about another's motivations or feelings are likely to be more effective than questions that leave out the 'think' component.

However, the following example indicates, that even with the precursor 'think' in place, there are occasions when this general rule might not be as effective. In the case presented here, the following utterance is complicated by the inclusion of a double layer of 'thinking' (from previously unpublished data).

Oak Clinic

```
Therapist   What d'you. think he thinks he's got out of being
            at ((names place))?
            (3.6)
Mother:     I d- I don't know really cos he h- he doesn't
            (0 2) say (0.4) he doesn't say a lot about here
```

Although the practitioner begins with a 'what do you think' question opening, they add a layer of complexity by asking what the other person thinks '*what do you think he thinks…*'. While the initial '*what do you think*' provides the recipient with the opportunity to speculate on a range of possible answers, the inclusion of considering what 'he thinks' also indicates that the speculated on other may have a range of possible motivations. Thus, it makes it tricky for the recipient of the question to hypothesise about which of those potential alternatives might be relevant. In other words, the addition of 'what do you think *he* thinks' opens up the recipient's options too broadly. Answering the question is made more difficult. The take-home learning therefore is that asking someone what they think about a situation is within their K+ arena of knowledge or knowledge hypothesis, but asking why something happened may not. Similarly, asking someone what they think about someone else's thoughts is also too far into the K− part of the spectrum of knowledge. This is evidenced by the fact that the recipient in this example struggles to provide an account for not knowing what someone else was thinking.

Negotiated Competency Expectations

Practitioners and adult family members alike have implicit expectations about who might have greater knowledge of certain topics than others. This is typically displayed in relation to who questions are addressed to. For example, if a question is addressed to a certain person, this is a display of an expectation that the recipient is in a K+ position to be able to answer that question. Recipient selection can be accomplished either by addressing the person by name or by eye gaze (see Sacks et al., 1974). While recipient selection is an indicator of the speaker's expectations of the competency of the selected person to be able to answer the question, sometimes other parties may display alternative competency expectations. An example of this may be when a child is asked a question by the practitioner, but the parent steps in to answer the question on behalf of the child. In such cases, while the practitioner displays an expectation that the child has competency to answer, the parent's interjection indicates an expectation that the child may not be able to answer or to answer fully. In other words, the child's K+ position is interactionally negotiated and accomplished through a dynamic series of turns (from previously unpublished data).

Family 20

```
Clin Psy     Have you tried anything to try and (1) deal
             with that?
             (1.4)
Clin Psy     Or has a- have you tried anything that
             worked or you?
             (6.0)
Mum          (It's you not us)
             (1.0)
Mum          She ha- she has=
Clin Psy     =Any strategies you u[se,]
Mum                                [Sh]e says she has urges to
             pick up people's books and drop 'em and she
             clenches her fists don't you?
```

The clinical psychologist directs a question to the child to ask what strategies they use to manage their behaviour. After a short pause (1.4 seconds), the psychologist tries the question again and waits for the child to answer. After 6 seconds, the mother prompts the child that there is an expectation they answer the question and not the parents '*it's you, not us*'. Eventually when the child does not offer an answer to the question, the mother answers on the child's behalf by showing that the child does indeed use strategies.

Importantly, it is not always the case that the parents treat the child as having competence to answer a question. In these instances, the practitioner may display an assumption of a child's competency or K+ position in relation to a particular topic about themselves, but this is contested or resisted by other family members. The following data example illustrates the complexity of negotiating subjective knowledge (from previously unpublished data).

6 Children's Competence

Family 1

```
MHN      WHEN did those thoughts s↓tart?
Child    °bout-° (0.54) two month ago
MHN      Okay-
Mum      be a bit longer than that now w↓on't [↑it?
Child                                         [No no not when
         I's th↑inking bad th↓ings
Mum      ↑Yeah probably about three month
```

The practitioner in this sequence asked a question of the child that apparently was expected to be within their scope of K+ competency; the child's *'thoughts'*. The response is a clear and relevant answer of about *'two month ago'*, which is acknowledged and accepted by the practitioner. However, the mother then interjected to disagree with the child's assessment and provided an alternative answer, arguing it to be *'a bit longer'*. The tag question *'won't it?'* invited the child to agree with her reformulation, and despite the child's emphatic retaining of the original answer, the mother nonetheless reiterated her perspective that the child's answer was incorrect. Although knowledge about the child's thoughts might be reasonably anticipated to be within the child's scope of K+ knowledge, the mother in this example asserted that her competency to know the child's thoughts was more valid than her child's. In other words, she claims a higher K+ position about the child's thoughts than the child has. This is a good example of how competency is not something to be thought of as intrinsic to a person (i.e., that they do or do not have it), but demonstrates clearly that competency is a contextually situated and dynamically accomplished achievement between practitioners, parents, and children.

> Children's anticipated competency is demonstrated by practitioners in the questions they ask children to answer. However, parents may disagree, dispute or present alternative answers which demonstrate that children's competency is contextually and dynamically negotiated.

Final Thoughts

In this chapter, we have illustrated that competency is fluid and dynamic, it is negotiated and situated. While there is clearly an aspect of a child's competency that is connected to their developmental and chronological age, much of their competency is situated in relation to their anticipated domains of knowledge. In other words, internal states, such as thoughts, feelings, memories, perceptions, beliefs, experiences, attitude, and values, are presumed to be more within the child's domain of knowledge than other people's, including family members. In this chapter, we have talked about K+ in reference to a greater knowledge competency in a particular area, in contrast with K- where there is a lesser knowledge competency in a particular area. The data we have provided in this chapter have demonstrated that expectations of subjective knowledge are negotiated between practitioners and family members. In the following practitioner voice box, Box 6.3, Olga Smoliak describes how children's competency might be negotiated and managed in her professional relationships with children and families.

> **Box 6.3 Practitioner Voice, Olga Smoliak**
>
> Practitioner voices
> Olga Smoliak
> Associate professor, psychologist, and therapist
>
>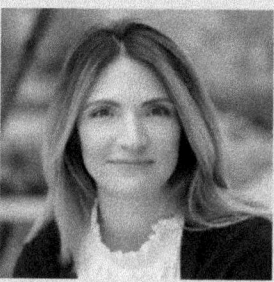
>
> Olga Smoliak, PhD, is an Associate Professor in Family Relations and Applied Nutrition at the University of Guelph, Canada. She is also a clinical/

(continued)

Box 6.3 (continued)

counselling psychologist and marriage and family therapist. Her primary research areas are postmodern (discursive) therapies and research (discursive psychology, conversation analysis, critical discourse analysis). She co-edited *Therapy as Discourse: Research and Practice* (with T. Strong) and *The Handbook of Counselling and Psychotherapy* in Canada.

As a clinical psychologist and family therapist, I find the notion of competence as interactionally claimed and negotiated (rather than static or inherent to people) as highly relevant to professional practice. To this end, the chapter sensitised me to how knowledge in specific domains can be distributed among family members and between professionals and clients. Of note, a few points stood out for me. I learned that many professionals tend to treat children as less competent than adults. An interactional lens on competence encourages practitioners to determine the child's (in)competence *through* inquiry rather than presuming it beforehand. Practitioners can also ensure that they avoid assuming that the child lacks knowledge, while also allowing the child to claim ignorance (e.g., "You may not know the answer, but I wanted to ask..." or "It's ok if you don't know, but...").

The chapter also highlighted how assumptions of competence can be negotiated between family members. Indeed, some family members may routinely position themselves as more knowledgeable compared to other family members and speak on behalf of other family members. For example, a parent may presume their child's lesser competence and position themselves as more competent in discussing a specific matter. Professionals can, therefore, attend to how family members position themselves and each other as more or less knowledgeable and invite redistribution of knowledge within the family (e.g., by amplifying views of family members positioned as less competent). For example, a professional does not need to automatically endorse or join the parent's positioning of the child and can instead reposition the child as competent or a legitimate informant.

Finally, the chapter stresses that competence is not unidimensional but rather multifaceted or domain-specific (e.g., the child may be knowledgeable in one area and less knowledgeable in another area). This more nuanced view of competence implies that professionals not only share expertise with clients but can learn from clients, including children. Likewise, children can be informed about matters outside of their knowledge domain (e.g., aims and nature of professional encounters, parents' concerns). Overall, the chapter offers a unique understanding of competence in the context of professional encounters that can benefit practitioners seeking to improve their practice.

Therapeutically speaking, sometimes parents habitually invalidate their children's reports about their internal or subjective experiences of thoughts, feelings, and perceptions of events, by correcting or disagreeing. In effect, the parent is disputing the child's K+ position in relation to their own personal knowledge. While this may be valid in relation to objective facts, such as the child's age, when it relates to subjective matters like thoughts, feelings, beliefs, and opinions, 'correcting' a child has the effect of minimising or invalidating the child's confidence in their K+ position regarding internal states. As a practitioner working with families, it may be helpful to notice parent and child interactions where these kind of competency disputes occur. Noticing how parents treat their child as competent or incompetent is useful familial understanding for the practitioner. Such interjections from parents can be informative for understanding the family dynamic, and different family member positioning. This has important implications for the child's beliefs about their own competencies in different knowledge domains. We summarise the key messages from the chapter in Box 6.4.

> **Box 6.4 Key Points**
>
> - Competence is interactionally situated.
> - Social norms dictate that there are typical scripts for different contexts or situations.
> - The K+ K– knowledge continuum can be used to illustrate anticipated knowledge domains.
> - Professional knowledge includes specific language and vocabulary, which may be less familiar to children and their families.
> - Normatively, children and adults are treated as having competency to report on their own thoughts and feelings; however, knowledge about the thoughts and feelings of others can only be inferred.
> - In professional interactions with children and families, children's competency is negotiated.
> - Consistent competency invalidation may undermine children's confidence.

References

Bateman, A., & Church, A. (2016). Children's knowledge-in-interaction: An introduction. In A. Bateman & A. Church (Eds.), *Children's knowledge-in-interaction: Studies in conversation analysis* (pp. 1–12). Springer.

Bone, C., O'Reilly, M., Karim, K., & Vostanis, P. (2014). "They're not witches…": Young children and their parents' perceptions and experiences of child and adolescent mental health services. *Child: Care, Health, and Development, 41*(3), 450–458.

Burman, E. (2008). *Developments: Child, image, nation*. Routledge.

Clemente, I. (2009). Progressivity and participation: Children's management of parental assistance in paediatric chronic pain encounters. *Sociology of Health and Illness, 31*(6), 872–888.

Danby, S. (2002). The communicative competence of young children. *Australian Journal of Early Childhood, 27*(3), 25–30.

Edwards, D. (1995). Two to tango: Script formulations, dispositions, and rhetorical symmetry in relationship troubles talk. *Research on Language and Social Interaction, 28*(4), 319–350.

Edwards, D. (1994). Script formulations: An analysis of event descriptions in conversation. *Journal of Language and Social Psychology, 13*(3), 211–247.

Heritage, J. (2012). Epistemics in action: Action formation and territories of knowledge. *Research on Language and Social Interaction, 45*, 1–29.

Hutchby, I., & Moran-Ellis, J. (1998). Situating children's competence. In I. Hutchby & J. Moran-Ellis (Eds.), *Children and social competence: Arenas of social action* (pp. 7–26). The Falmer Press.

Hutchby, I., & O'Reilly, M. (2010). Children's participation and the familial moral order in family therapy. *Discourse Studies, 12*(1), 49–64.

Kuczynski, L. (2003). Beyond bidirectionality: Bilateral conceptual frameworks for understanding dynamics in parent-child relations. In L. Kuczynski (Ed.), *Handbook of dynamics in parent-child relations* (pp. 1–24). Sage.

Masterpasqua, F. (1989). A competence paradigm for psychological practice. *American Psychologist, 44*(11), 1366–1371.

O'Reilly, M. (2008). 'What value is there in children's talk?' Investigating family therapist's interruptions of parents and children during the therapeutic process. *Journal of Pragmatics, 40*, 507–524.

O'Reilly, M., Hutchby, I., & Kiyimba, N. (2019). Children's competence in assessments. In J. Lamerichs, S. Danby, A. Bateman, & S. Ekberg (Eds.), *Children's social competence in mental health talk*. Palgrave Macmillan.

O'Reilly, M., Lester, J. N., & Muskett, T. (2016). Children's claims to knowledge regarding their mental health experiences and practitioners' negotiation of the problem. *Patient Education and Counseling [Special Issue], 99*, 905–910.

Ortega, F. (2009). The cerebral subject and the challenge of neurodiversity. *BioSocieties, 4*, 425–445.

Plaza Lara, C. (2016). The competence paradigm in education applied to the multicomponent models of translator competences. *Journal of Translator Education and Translation Studies, 1*(2), 4–19.

Sacks, H. (1992). In G. Jefferson (Ed.), *Lectures on conversation* (Vol. I & II). Basil Blackwell.

Sacks, H., Schegloff, E., & Jefferson, G. (1974). A simplest systematics for the organization of turn-taking for conversation. *Language, 50*(4), 696–735.

Schaarschmidt, T. (2018). The art of lying. *The Scientific American.* from https://www.scientificamerican.com/article/the-art-of-lying/

Sodian, B., Kristen-Antonow, S., & Kloo, D. (2020). How does children's theory of mind become explicit? A review of longitudinal findings. *Child Development Perspectives, 14*(3), 171–177.

Stafford, V., Hutchby, I., Karim, K., & O'Reilly, M. (2016). "Why are you here?" Seeking children's accounts of their presentation to CAMHS. *Clinical Child Psychology and Psychiatry, 21*(1), 3–18.

Stivers, T. (2012). Physician–child interaction: When children answer physicians' questions in routine medical encounters. *Patient Education and Counseling, 87*(1), 3–9.

Stivers, T. (2001). Negotiating who presents the problem: Next speaker selection in pediatric encounters. *Journal of Communication, 51*(2), 1–31.

Theobald, M. (2016). Achieving competence: The interactional features of children's storytelling. *Childhood, 23*(1), 87–104.

Wellman, H. (1990). *The child's theory of mind.* MIT.

Part III

Attending to the Different Needs of Family Members

7

Managing Age-Appropriate Conversations with Children Present

Learning Objectives

- Consider when certain topics of conversation may be inappropriate for children to be party to
- Recognise the potential negative impact on children where parents may speak derogatively about them in their presence
- Identify the benefits of short periods of separating children from adults in the clinical conversation
- Critically reflect on the ways in which conversations with different combinations of family members might be accomplished

Introduction

When working with families and engaging families in conversation, one of the challenges is to negotiate appropriate topics of conversation with children present. Although what constitutes an appropriate topic of conversation may vary between cultures, there are usually normative ideas about what constitute adult topics that are not suitable for children to overhear or be engaged in. In this chapter, we utilise empirical data to explore some of the problems involved in navigating this challenging endeavour. Drawing on our family therapy and mental health assessment data where the practitioner attempts to establish the nature of the difficulties within the family, we highlight the value of having periods of time where parents and children have opportunities to present their versions of events separately. This potentially negates the troublesome situation of parents speaking pejoratively about their children in front of their children.

Appropriate Topics of Conversation

While the concepts of childhood and adolescence as socially constructed have changed over time, and are culturally tied, there are normative expectations about differences in the appropriateness of 'adult' and 'child' topics of conversation. From a maturational perspective, children of different ages become incrementally aware of the adult world through observation, education, digital media, peer influence, and a range of other influences. There is a common presumption that it is part of the adult responsibility to protect children from not only the physical risks in their environment but also exposure to information that is beyond their developmental maturity. For example, young children should be protected from certain topics of conversation, such as sex (Hutchby & Moran-Ellis, 1998). In mental health settings, one reason why a family may be involved in support (like therapy) is that there may have been abuse or intimate partner violence. The children themselves may even have been victims of abuse and so conversations about what would normally be adult topics may need to involve children in these situations but require delicate handling. There are, of course, numerous different ways this may happen, and multiple possible topics of conversation that could be defined as developmentally inappropriate.

By way of example, we present a series of extracts from our family therapy data with one specific family over several sessions. The series of conversations relate to the father's brother who was previously convicted of a child sex offence. The discussion in the current therapy relates to the appropriateness of talking about this offence in front of the children. The following extract is from the sixth session and present were both parents and one of the three children (the youngest aged six years) (taken from

7 Managing Age-Appropriate Conversations with Children...   177

O'Reilly & Parker, 2014, p. 294, and an example we return to later in our discussion of risk and risk assessment).

Clamp family

```
Dad:   she <turned round> and told my brother <in front of the
       three children> (.) <that 'e cannot 'ave anythin' t' do
       wiv ↑my children because 'e 'as sex with children>
FT:    ↓Right
```

In this example, the father complains to the therapist that the social worker ('she') on a visit to their home had expressed to his brother that he should not have contact with the children because of his previous conviction. The father's complaint mainly relates to his report of the social worker using inappropriate language in front of his *'three children'*, that is, that his brother *'has sex with children'*. The following extract is taken from later in the same session, where the mother corroborates the information provided from the father about the social worker (from O'Reilly & Parker, 2014, p. 296).

Clamp family

```
FT:    that actually <social services> would like him out the ↑way
Dad;   That's what she turned round [and told 'im in front of
       the kids
Mum:                                 [Yes (.) that's what Joan Karr
       ↑told 'im (.) she told 'im t' <get out of the house>
```

When the family therapist seeks clarification about the incident, the father reiterates his account of what the social worker had *'turned round* and told 'im'* in front of his children about his brother. (*turned round is an English colloquialism to indicate an unexpected interjection). His wife corroborates the account by specifically naming the social worker and adding to the narrative that she ordered the children's uncle to leave the house.

These two examples are illustrations of parents indicating what are appropriate or inappropriate topics of conversation for practitioners to have in the presence of children. Problematically, in narrating their complaint about the social worker to the family therapist, the parents do so in front of their six-year-old child who is also present within the therapy session. Although it is beyond the scope of the family therapist in the current session to address what did or did not happen in the family home, as they cannot go back in time to prevent the child from hearing that information, there is scope for the therapist to have some influence over what topics are given floor space in the current interaction. The following example demonstrates that this is what the therapist did within this session (taken from O'Reilly & Parker, 2014, p. 299).

Clamp family

```
FT:     ↑Can I jus' (.) is it ↑alright for us t' >talk
        about this<
Dad:    ↑Not really not with Ronald being ↓'ere
((8 lines of talk omitted for readability))
FT:     Right (.) can I? (.) >I mean I it< [sounds like quite
        an <important conversation>
Mum:                                       [He said (.) if ↑we'd
        give ↓'im
Dad:    ↓Hu::m
FT:     can I ask if = see if <one of my colle:agues> could ↑sit
Dad:    ↑Yeah
FT:     with (.) with Ronald and er::m
Dad:    ↑Yeah
FT:     Cuz I'm not sure 'e should hear ↑this
```

Once the family therapist realises that the topic of conversation has moved towards something that could be deemed as inappropriate for children to listen to, he raises his concern with the parents. Indeed, he asks *'is it alright for us to talk about this?'*. The father takes the opportunity to affirm that the topic is inappropriate for his son and the therapist moves to suggest that one of his *'colleagues'* takes the child out of the session and sits with him, so that the parents can continue and talk more freely with the therapist about the incident. We have shared this example to show one way that topics of conversation such as this might be managed. Fortunately, in this situation, there was a member of staff available to sit with the child so that the therapist and parents could continue their conversation without him present. However, this was not always possible, as the following example illustrates. Here, in session eight with the same family, the same topic is raised again, but this time there was not a member of staff available to take the child out of the session. Following a session with just the parents (session seven), the therapist invited the uncle to attend session eight. Although Joe, the uncle did attend session eight, due to problems with arranging childcare for their son, the parents also brought Ronald the six-year-old. Problematically, a session that had been planned to have an adult conversation with the parents and the uncle became one where the child was also present.

Clamp family (from previously unpublished data)

```
FT:     Right (2.0) what what do you think abo::ut the stuff we
        talked about last time (.) do we leave that?
Mum:    ↓Yeah
FT:     Okay (.) what do you think Joe?
Joe:    I don't really know (.) I'll talk [about
        anything I will
Mum:                                      [Heh heh heh heh
FT:     Well I guess that sort of conversation's gonna be
        pretty difficult for you anyway (3.5) ok↑ay er::m (.)
        sounds like everybody's saying (3.0) we can do this
        next time
Dad:    >Yeah I think so< 'cause he don't understand anyway but
        (.) whatever like you know
        (1.0)
FT:     Yeah but I don' think it's be appropri[ate to talk
        about it
```

> Notably, the interlocutors within the interaction determined the appropriateness of the topic, rather than us as analysts.

> **Box 7.1 Reflective activity on Types of Conversations**
>
> Reflective activity
>   Types of conversations
>   In your professional context when working with families, consider what topics of conversation might be important to talk about without children present. Consider how you might negotiate those decisions with adult family members.
>   This is important to think about carefully, as while the decision is likely to be navigated with the parents, it still does involve the child and so there will need to be some engagement of the child in managing the situation of leaving the room (e.g., you may need to persuade them or offer them toys to play with).

This extract illustrates the conversation had occurred regarding what they can or cannot talk about. It appears that the therapist is tactfully suggesting that talking about the sex offence would not be appropriate with a child present. Within conversation analysis, the term recipient design is used to express the way that speakers construct what they say as appropriate for the person they are speaking to (Sacks & Schegloff, 1979). He does so initially by suggesting *'do we leave that?'* and after seeking confirmation from the uncle summarises *'sounds like everybody's saying we can do this next time'*. When the father indicates that it may be okay to continue with the conversation because the child does not *'understand anyway'*, the therapist takes a clearer stance by stating *'I don't think it's be appropriate to talk about it'*. While the practitioner working with this family seeks to make the decision collaboratively, ultimately, they take responsibility for the child's wellbeing in the current session. At this point, we invite you to try the reflective activity in Box 7.1.

Talking About the Child, with the Child Present

In mental health conversations with families, there is often the need to gather information from parents about their children's difficulties to assess clinical need and possible support or interventions that may be required. Typically, however, due to practical circumstances such as children attending appointments with their parents or being present in the home environment, the children may be able to overhear the comments that their parents make about them to the practitioner. A dilemma occurs therefore for practitioners between ascertaining full and accurate information about the child's problems and managing the appropriateness of what children may overhear.

When someone is talking about another person who is not present in a negative or derogatory way, we tend to refer to this in mundane conversations as gossiping. In our earlier research, we extended this concept to professional contexts to include a form of institutional gossiping where parents talk about their children in pejorative ways in front of them (Parker & O'Reilly, 2012). We acknowledge that the term 'gossiping' is not one that is usually considered to be part of professional interactions with families. Perhaps a more usual terminology that might be used in mental health interactions would be overhearing, yet it does share some features with mundane gossip. This includes, that gossip is negative, remedial, triadic, and often sanctioned. In fact, in family therapy for example, where the practitioner is speaking to one family member in the presence of other family members, the practitioner might ask other family members what it is like to 'overhear' that conversation.

When children who are present are talked about in a derogatory way, it has implications for the appropriateness or therapeutic value of them hearing explicit criticism and invalidation from their parents. Before we introduce some data examples of children being talked about, we present a short extract where the male therapist and the husband are talking about the wife in her presence and actually used the term 'gossiping' to conceptualise the nature of that talk (taken from Parker & O'Reilly, 2012, p. 461).

Webber family

```
FT:    Mandy, [I'm gonna talk t' you cuz =
Mum:          [↑Yeah
FT:    = you've be:en sat very patiently lis[tenin' t' =
Mum:                                         [It's alright
FT:    = what t' what t- two men 'ave be:en sayin' (0.4) e::rm
       almost <about you> and almost like we're gossipin'
Mum:   Heh heh heh
FT:    gossipin' in front of you e::rm
```

In this extract, the family therapist orients to how it might feel for the wife to listen to two men talking about her without including her in the conversation. By positioning himself and the husband as *'men'*, he acknowledges that there has been a degree of exclusion of the wife from that aspect of the conversation and that she has been the topic of their conversation. Thus, the therapist conceptualises this conversation as having the qualities of gossip *'almost like we're gossiping in front of you'*. The use of the phrase *'in front of you'* is an explicit acknowledgement of her presence, in contrast to gossip that would normally occur behind someone's back. In family groups where children tend to hold a less powerful position, there are fewer opportunities for children to defend themselves, and furthermore there is a greater risk of emotional harm to overhear their parents characterising them in negative ways due to developmental vulnerability. We provide two examples of parental negative appraisals (taken from Parker & O'Reilly, 2012, p. 464).

Niles family

```
Dad:    <we've got t' sort> (.) o:r get some medication or
        somet t' calm 'is temper ↓down (.) cuz 'e's ↑schizo
```

Webber family

```
Mum:    >Yer know< ↑so we've got (0.2) small kids either <side
        of us> ↑now haven't we? (0.2) an' they're in the garden
        it's (0.4) it's like the scho:ol said 'e's like a
        preda↑tor
```

Taken from different families, these two examples show different ways in which parents used extreme and stigmatising labels to characterise their children, *'schizo'* and *'predator'*. Problematically, in a non-institutional context, where mental health labels are used in this pejorative way, they would be considered insults. Moving beyond purely describing the children's behaviour for the sake of the therapeutic business, the parents use pejorative terms about their children in front of them. Although these extreme formulations may serve an institutional purpose of demonstrating a need for mental health services, they simultaneously undermine the child who is in the same room and may negatively impact on the child's sense of self-worth.

7 Managing Age-Appropriate Conversations with Children... 183

Regardless of how parents may talk about or to their children in their home environment, in an institutional context it is the practitioner who is required to take responsibility for modelling and managing more appropriate language. The following two extracts are examples where the practitioner attempts to re-include talked about children in the conversation and orients to the difficulty, they may be experiencing of hearing their parents talk in negative ways about them (taken from Parker & O'Reilly, 2012, p. 469).

Clamp family

```
FT:   we did a lot of talkin' abo::ut (0.8)some of the things
      that you do (.) that your mum and dad aren't too happy
      about and I guess I jus' wanted t' say that I know that
      it's re:ally difficult t' sit there and ↑listen
```

Here, the practitioner expects that it may be difficult or uncomfortable for the child to listen to the negative evaluations about him from his parents. He recognises that the adults in the room have been talking about the child about *'the things that you do'*, which he frames quite broadly, and in so doing recognises that these things might be *'difficult to sit there and listen'* to by the child. Similarly, in the following extract, the practitioner acknowledges the potential discomfort for the child of listening in to a conversation between adults about him (taken from Parker and O'Reilly, 2012, p. 469).

Webber family

```
FT:    >I know that< you're looking uneasy already Da(h)niel
Mum:   Heh he[h heh
```

Another tool for practitioners is to be attentive to visual cues such as body language when assessing the impact of difficult conversations on children who are present. In this extract, the practitioner comments to the child that he is *'looking uneasy'* as a precursor to an invitation to explain how he is feeling.

In both extracts, the therapist orients to the delicacy of the topic at hand. As Silverman and Peräkylä (1990) have highlighted in their work, typically in a therapeutic conversation where delicate topics of

> **Box 7.2 Reflective Activity on Using the Tools in Your Practice**
>
> Reflective activity
>   Using tools
>   In the previous extracts, we have shown three ways that practitioners might seek to re-include children in conversations about them to check that they are okay, to invite their point of view, and to confirm facts. These were:
>
> - Use an open question to invite the child to comment on the process of hearing parents' descriptions.
> - Use a closed question to propose the likely discomfort or difficulty for the child.
> - Comment on visual cues indicating discomfort to invite verbalisation of that discomfort.
>
> In each of these cases, the practitioner comments on metaprocesses of the interaction rather than the content of the conversation. We invite you to reflect on how you might use one or more of these tools in your own professional context to manage difficult multi-party conversations with children present.

conversation are raised, speakers tend "to orient to and make use of the socially and culturally prescribed etiquette of approaching a delicate issue" (p. 303). At this point, we invite you to try the reflective activity in Box 7.2.

Negotiating Time with Parents and Children Separately

As we have seen from the previous two sections, there are great benefits to having all family members present at the same time in a mental health setting. However, children's presence in adult conversations can at times be quite problematic. Additionally due to the adult–child power imbalance in these interactions, it may be difficult for children to freely articulate their own perspectives with parents present. Therefore, there is value in having opportunities for parents and children to have a conversation with the practitioner separately at various junctures in the process.

The Value of Separation

There are various reasons why negotiating time with parents and children separately can be beneficial including:

- Opportunity to discuss adult topics with adult family members without children present.
- Protecting children from hearing adult family members reporting behaviours and events concerning their children in negative ways.
- Opportunity for either adults or children to talk about sensitive or difficult things in a more confidential space.
- Children can present their version of events freely without concern about parental contradiction.
- Protecting children from seeing their parents upset or angry about their difficulties.
- Opportunity to assess for risk or safeguarding issues.
- Opportunity to discuss how parents coordinate their parenting efforts (or not) regarding the discussion item of concern pertaining to their child.

The following two extracts demonstrate the respective value to both the parents and children to having time apart to speak to a mental health practitioner separately. In the first extract, the therapist articulates the benefits of why some time without the child present might be useful, which is supported by the mother who recognises the usefulness of being able to speak freely.

Family 18 (from previously unpublished data)

```
Therapist      as we were sayin' because it is that age ↓really
               and (.) we thought actually it ↓might be much
               better (.) [for]
Mum                       [Yeah]
Therapist      (0.59) for both of you ↓really [(    )]
               separate (.) =
Mum                                           [Yeah]
Therapist      = ↓er: space and [>(I was thinking that)<] some
               things might be very difficult to dis↓cuss
Mum                             [Ye:ah that's fine]
               An' not o[nly th]at it's not very ↓nice for (name)
               to hear negativity all the ↓time is it?
Therapist               [Um:]
```

In this example, the therapist indicates that there is a benefit to both the child and the parent in having separate time. In proposing the separate space, the therapist also offers a reason for why this might be beneficial, by proposing that *'some things might be very difficult to discuss'*. The mother agrees with this idea and further adds a secondary reason why separate conversations could be useful, by recognising that *'it's not very nice for N to hear negativity all the time'*. By using naturally occurring data like this, as practitioners we can learn some exemplars of good practice. Apart from offering adult family members the opportunity to talk freely about their struggles with their children, it can be very valuable to provide children, especially in adolescent years, the opportunity to articulate their version of events.

> An example of good practice is in three parts: recognising the potential need or value of separate conversations with adult and child family members, offering a potential reason, and collaborating with the family members to finalise a plan of action.

In the following extract (taken from Parker, 2003, p. 138), the adolescent male reveals to the therapist the ways in which his parents behave towards him in his home setting that are not evident in the institutional interaction.

Gallagher House

```
Client:      You don't see how they tre̱at me.
             (2)
Client:      Js- na̱sty really na̱sty.
             (1.2)
Client:      How they can just (1.6) s- swe̱ar at me and, (1)
             threaten to kic̆k my head in an-, (1.4) and [then
             just be as nice as- nice as ↑ pie, =
Therapist:                                              [(I've
             not seen that today)
Client:      = to my sisters.
             (5.4)
```

((17 lines omitted))

```
Client:      They keep pulling that back up, oh when he was
             little he couldn't of loved you more. Y- w- (0.2) He
             couldn't have loved anybody more than he loved you.
             ((feigned deep voice))
             (0.6)
Client:      (Well) it's a shame that I can't remember none of
             that an I can remember is him pu̱nching me, an-
             (0.4) shou̱tin' at me and swearing at me an-
             (4.2)
```

This extract begins with the adolescent *'you don't see how they treat me'*. By having time separate from his parents to talk to the practitioner, the adolescent can speak more freely about what goes on at home 'behind closed doors'. He argues that his father *'swears', 'threatens' 'punches'* and *'shouts'* at him but is *'as nice as pie'* to his sisters (meaning he acts pleasantly towards the sisters). It is important that the adolescent is provided with the opportunity to disclose these kinds of behaviours, because, as the therapist recognises, these things are not always revealed or evident in the clinic room *'I've not seen that today'*. Potentially, this practitioner is highlighting the difference between what the adolescent is saying and what she has seen herself and may imply that she might doubt the validity of his claims. From a safeguarding perspective, however, it is important as practitioners to take note of and carefully consider claims like this as there may be a need to take further action to protect the child or adolescent.

> Time alone with children can provide a useful opportunity to ascertain if there is any risk.

While the possibility of talking to children and adults separately might be proposed early in a session, the implementation of that separation will vary according to context and to the specific in situ conversation. Broadly speaking, the strategy for separate conversations might be proactive or reactive. The previous extracts were examples of proactive decisions on the part of the practitioner to provide the opportunity for parents and children to speak separately about their concerns. The following extract demonstrates the value of being sensitive to the course of the interaction and using separation reactively to care for the needs of all family members in the moment. In this example (previously unpublished data), the mother in the family began to cry as she recalled the death of her son, and this was the catalyst for the practitioners suggesting the need to talk separately from the daughter.

Family 12

```
Nurse        Obviously we spoke to ↓mum a:nd mum gave us the:
             (0.26) the sort of sa:me (0.39) incidences that
             she's (.) e[xplained] to you
Asst Psych              [Ye:ah]
Nurse        (0.62) Um: she also told us (.) in quite a lot of
             detail about her brother
Asst Psych   Ye:ah
Nurse        So w- we had to split ↓up coz mum was [quite
             up]set =
Asst Psych                                         [YEah]
Nurse        and [I thi]nk it would've been upsetting =
Asst Psych       [Yeah]
Nurse        = for her to see her mum get u[pset]
Asst Psych                                 [well I was] quite
             sur↓prised that she still remembered (.) couple
             because she's only ↓what three wasn't she ↑three
             four when he died
Nurse        he di:ed in two thousand and seven
```

What this extract demonstrates, is that the intention to separate the mother and child for discussion was to give the mother space to talk about her grief without the daughter seeing her mother upset. The nurse orients to the possible detrimental impact on the child by framing the reason for separation as being '*upsetting*' to witness her mother '*get upset*'. However, there were benefits for the child as well as the child remembered quite a lot of detail despite being a young age when her brother died, which provided a space for her to also connect with her grief.

Techniques for Separation

In this next section, our focus is on offering potential ways for practitioners to negotiate time with parents without the children present, and likewise, time with the child or children without the parents present. In so doing, we recognise that this will not necessarily be appropriate in all circumstances and clinical judgement will need to be exercised accounting the unique aspects of the work. There are different ways to introduce the topic with families of taking some time out to speak separately. In the following extract (from previously unpublished data), we demonstrate one technique which is to normalise the process as part of the usual institutional business.

Family 1

```
MHN      (.hhh) What we were think↓ing before you came up was
         that (.) pa:rt way through this what we usually do is
         split ↓up (0.87) er:m so I'll have a chat with ↓you if
         that's okay, (0.35) erm (.) and then Dr V(name) wi:ll
         (.) speak to your mum ab↓out (.) the kind of things
         like when you were a ba↓by and s↓tuff (0.74) e:rm
         (0.42) ↑is that okay with ↑yo↓u and then we can talk
         (.) a bit more about (.) coz it ↑sounds ↓like there's
         quite a lot going ↑on for ↓you doesn't ↓it really
Mum      yeah there is- it's quite dist↓urbing ↓really
```

This extract demonstrates a simple technique which is to highlight at the beginning of a session with a family that the practitioner would like to take some time later to talk separately. This is accomplished by using the phrase *'what we usually do is'*, which normalises the suggestion and indicates that this is routine rather than specifically identifying this family as uniquely needing something different. In this example, the nurse using a minimal confirmation seeking question within his discourse, *'is that okay with you'* whereas other practitioners may take more time to collaborate with families and ensure their cooperation. The following extract is an example of this. Notably, in the previous extract the practitioner highlights at the beginning of the session the likelihood of this happening later. The following extract (from previously unpublished data) demonstrates the actual implementation of the separation later in a session.

Family 18

```
Doctor       So probably it'd be: good if we: could (0.41)
             split you and mum ↑up and (.) have a chat (0.44) so
             I will speak to ↑you
Child        Umhum
Doctor       Okay
             (0.21)
             and (name) will speak to ↑mum (.) is that alright
             with you that ↓format?
Mum          Yeah [fine]
Doctor            >[Um jus' so] there's< jus' it gives you more
             space t' talk about your(0.31)>problems< cause
             sometimes it's ↓you know it not easy t' do would
             you be happy with ↓that an y[ou wo]uld you feel (.)
             you comfortable with ↓that
Child                                   [Yeah]
             °yeah°
Doctor       ↑Yeah and you okay with ↓that a[s well]
Mum                                          [Umhum]
             °Yeah (.) [no] problem°
Doctor                 [↑yeah]
             Is that is that fine ↓ (name)?
Therapist    I think yes [yes shall we]
Doctor                   [I think that would probably be th]e way
             to (0.52)
Therapist    Shall we meet in about half an hour
```

7 Managing Age-Appropriate Conversations with Children...

```
Doctor      HAlf an hour (0.35) f- forty minutes ↑time
Mum         °Yeah°
Doctor      ↑Yeah (.) so I'll spend some time with ↓you (0.41)
            an:d you can spend some time [with] °(name) yeah°
            can you take the ↓notes I'll just take down
            notes an'
```

Here the psychiatrist takes some time to ensure that the child is comfortable with the suggestion to meet separately and confirms this is acceptable with the mother. The key characteristics of implementing this technique were:

- The practitioner suggested separating.
- The potential benefits of talking separately were briefly outlined.
- Agreement and confirmation were established with the family members.
- A time frame was provided for how long the separate conversation would be.
- Clarification was made regarding which practitioner would be talking with which family member.

In addition to this list of strategies used just prior to different members of the family being separated to talk to different practitioners, it is worth bearing in mind that there may be further considerations relevant to rejoining the whole family group after this separation time. The main consideration noted from our data that the practitioner would negotiate with the separated family member was which aspects of their conversation would or would not be brought into the discussion with all reunited family members. For example, a child may disclose things in that separate conversation that they may not want the practitioner to repeat in front of their parents. Thus, we suggest from our data that good practice would be for practitioners to confirm with their client what things they would or would not like to be brought back into the room with the rest of the family.

Final Thoughts

In this chapter, we have addressed the important but complex matter of providing opportunity for all family members to discuss their concerns in a way that gives them freedom and space to do so, without negatively impacting other family members at the same time. We recognise that every family is different and negotiating what is best for all family members requires experience and skill to accomplish this successfully. Readers who are practitioners in the field of family mental health practice will be familiar with the challenges of multi-party, multi-generational work. Although this chapter has not been comprehensive in addressing all the factors involved in managing complex multi-party interactions, we have sought to highlight some of the key considerations. The two areas that we have focused on are the protection of children in the context of topics of conversation that may be inappropriate for children to be party to and in the context of adult family members speaking derogatively about them in their presence. Additionally, we have highlighted the potential benefits for practitioners to speak with adult and child family members separately to ascertain potential risk factors and to gather information from different perspectives. We have offered a couple of techniques that were identified in our data regarding how practitioners might initiate a suggestion of separate conversations with different family members. These are not the only ways of doing this, and we provide examples of data in this chapter by way of suggestion. We encourage you to reflect on how you have managed this endeavour in your own work, and how the ideas within this chapter might support your practice.

In the following practitioner voice box, Jenny Phaure discussed child-led therapy in the family-based therapy model.

In intergenerational multi-party conversations, it can be easy for the conversation to drift towards more of a focus on the interaction between adult practitioner and adult family members. There is always a risk of children being marginalised in these types of conversations and their needs to be inadvertently overlooked. What we have become aware of is the importance of practitioners consciously considering the child's voice, their wellbeing, and the impact of being party to negative discourse.

Box 7.3 Practitioner Voice, Jenny Phaure

Practitioner voices
Role family-based therapist
Jenny Phaure

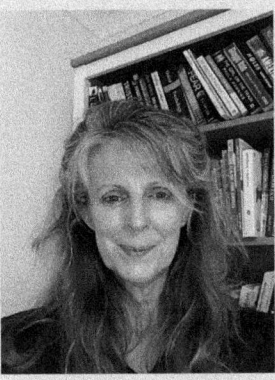

Jenny is a UK-based child and adolescent psychotherapist specialising in work with autistic children, young people, adults, and families.

The Family-Based Therapy Centre provides family-based therapy sessions alongside child, adult, and parent only sessions. The initial assessment is divided into 2 hours. Forty minutes of the first hour is initially alone with the child or young person (unless the child indicates that they would prefer one or both parents to remain). The remaining 20 minutes of the first hour is given over to a shared interactive game involving the child and parents. This affords the opportunity to observe parent–child interactions without the need for intrusive questions. With the focus on a third object, 'the game', there is a safety that enables family members to be themselves as much as possible. The therapist suggests a point at which the game may come to a natural pause, recognising the child's contribution, the child-focused hour comes to a natural close. The child/young person is invited to leave the session with another parent or safe person that may have accompanied them. If the session is conducted remotely, a more natural confidential space for the parent, only part of the session is more feasible where the child/young person remains in their own space with access to an activity nearby.

The child-led session is then followed by an hour with the parent(s). If it is not possible to complete 2 hours in one session, or if the child doesn't have access to a safe place or another supportive adult, then the second part of the session is organised at a time when there is space for the parents to speak freely and in confidence, usually during school time. In this way, the child/young person's voice is heard first and therefore reduces any

(continued)

> **Box 7.3** (continued)
>
> anticipatory anxiety that the child may be experiencing prior to the start of a session. A brief guide to how the initial assessment is going to be structured is sent out to parent's beforehand with a list of suggested items that the child/young person may like to bring to their part of the session. Suggested items include a special interest, creative activity that they enjoy, special item or book, an interactive game, and a sensory object or fidget that they use. The list of suggestions are items or objects that are centred in and around the child's world and of significance to them. This gesture anchors the family-based session around thinking about the child/young person's needs and begins to prepare the parent(s) as they also wonder with their child or young person about objects or items that have significance and meaning to them. This natural preparation acts as a gentle therapeutic technique for guiding how future sessions may progress.

> **Box 7.4 Key Points About Managing Togetherness and Separateness in Family Conversations**
>
> - Within most cultural contexts, there are normative expectations about certain topics of conversation that are considered 'adult' and therefore inappropriate for children to be exposed to.
> - Children are very sensitive to statements made by adult family members about their conduct and disposition and practitioners may play a role in supporting adults to not articulate derogatory statements about their children in front of them.
> - In mental health conversations with families, there are benefits in both talking with all family members together and benefits in talking with family members separately from one another.

Through analysis of interactions with mental health professionals and our own practice, we have come to appreciate the benefits of offering children space separate from their parents to talk about their feelings and concerns. Additionally, parents often benefit from time to talk freely to a practitioner without their child present so that they can fully articulate what is bothering them. We summarise the key messages from the chapter in Box 7.4.

References

Hutchby, I., & Moran-Ellis, J. (1998). Situating children's competence. In I. Hutchby & J. Moran-Ellis (Eds.), *Children and social competence: Arenas of social action* (pp. 7–26). The Falmer Press.

O'Reilly, M., & Parker, N. (2014). 'She needs a smack in the gob': Negotiating what is appropriate talk in front of children in family therapy. *Journal of Family Therapy, 36*(3), 287–307.

Parker, N. (2003). 'What do you think?': A discursive analysis of psychology in therapy talk. Doctoral thesis. Loughborough University.

Parker, N., & O'Reilly, M. (2012). 'Gossiping' as a social action in family therapy: The pseudo-absence and pseudo-presence of children. *Discourse Studies, 14*(4), 1–19.

Sacks, H., & Schegloff, E. (1979). Two preferences in the organization of reference to persons in conversation and their interaction. In G. Psathas (Ed.), *Everyday language: Studies in ethnomethodology* (pp. 15–21). Irvington.

Silverman, D., & Peräkylä, A. (1990). AIDS counselling: The interactional organisation of talk about 'delicate' issues. *Sociology of Health & Illness, 12*(3), 293–318.

8

Avoiding Shame and Blame

> **Learning Objectives**
>
> - Recognise the implications of blame and shame as a potential barrier to families accessing services
> - Critically assess the historical context that has shaped our understanding of parent blaming
> - Identify the ways in which families may use language to manage blame and accountability
> - Reflect on dichotomous accounting practices and establish a dialectic alternative

Introduction

The focus of this chapter is on blame and shame. There are many kinds of interactions that occur *between* family members and blaming others in the family for their difficulties may be one of those social actions. This may be the result of a range of different responses to the emotional reactivity that inevitably occurs between family members. As these responses often occur in quite patterned ways, some family therapists have found helpful ways to support family members to move from these predictable reactive patterns to mindful ways of responding (Tomm et al., 2014).

However, our focus for this chapter is not so much an investigation of these kinds of problematic patterned blame and shame sequences of interactions between family members, but *towards* family members. We examine the ways in which family members, particularly parents, may find themselves being positioned as accountable for their children's difficulties by others in wider society, and potentially also by the mental health professionals supporting them.

To contextualise that conversation, we begin by considering the social construction of polarised concepts, such as 'good' and 'bad', or 'sick' and 'well', or 'normal' and 'abnormal', 'moral' and 'immoral', 'nature' and 'nurture', or 'conformist' and 'deviant'. We have argued throughout this book that concepts such as these are not static or predetermined but socially constructed and therefore the meaning and boundaries of these concepts are fluid and temporal. The notion of blaming only makes sense within the context of constructs that position certain people as 'bad', 'abnormal', or 'deviant'. Therefore, we invite the reader to hold this in mind as we discuss some of the literature around blame and shame as they relate to family interaction in the context of mental health. The challenge of creating polarised social discourses that position some people as acceptable and others as unacceptable is that it creates a separation between the self and others, referred to as 'othering'. Arguably, from a psychodynamic perspective the so-called bad that we perceive in others, is a projection of the 'bad' that we cannot tolerate within ourselves.

In this chapter, we illustrate through our extracts of family therapy data that within the context of professional mental health conversations with families, there are several binary propositions that are either explicitly or implicitly revisited. We outline several of these below, with an explanatory description of how these discursive resources function:

- Good versus bad—this explanatory framework draws on a moral heuristic to position behaviours within a dichotomous construct.
- Sick versus well—narratives of health versus ill health are normative medicalised points of reference to distinguish those who need treatment.
- Normal versus abnormal—these are socially constructed boundaries of society and therefore culturally, historically, and politically mediated discourses.

8 Avoiding Shame and Blame

- Moral versus immoral—these are socially constructed appraisals that legitimise the activity of making judgements to vindicate or condemn others.
- Nature versus nurture—aetiological explanations that contrast biological causal factors with environmental influences.
- Conformist versus deviant—unspoken social schemas dictate how people should behave, and when these are transgressed, it becomes legitimate to impose sanctions.

These polemic constructs are ubiquitously used in every family conversation, but because of their universality and the fact that they operate implicitly and subtly, they are not always immediately apparent. It may be helpful for practitioners to be mindful of how these discursive resources are drawn upon and articulated, particularly in contexts where blame and accountability are disputed. Supporting families to move away from mono-causal, black or white discourses about the causes of problems, involves helping them to consider the possibilities that both sides may have some truth in them. The illustration below demonstrates how this can be the case, where each person sees the number from their own perspective. Depending how you look at it, the number could be a six or a nine. Both are correct:

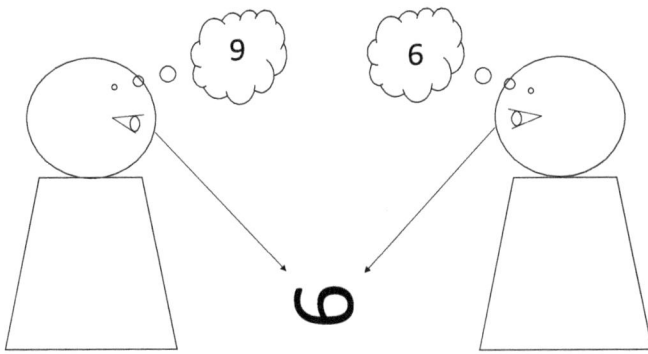

We suggest you think about your own practice context by engaging with the reflective activity in Box 8.1.

> **Box 8.1 Reflective Activity: Noticing Dichotomous Accounting Practices**
>
> Reflective activity
> Accounting practices
> Practitioners working in the field of mental health are likely familiar with the tendency for many clients to operate within a 'black and white' world view. The list of dichotomous discursive resources exemplifies ways in which this 'black and white' thinking might present itself in a family conversation. A therapeutic alternative to this polarisation of thinking is to adopt a dialectic approach. Dialectic means to consider that there is some truth in both ends of the spectrum. In other words, the phrase 'both/and' can be drawn upon rather than 'either/or'.
>
> - Consider ways in which a dialectic approach may be valuable in working with families who have this polarising kind of discursive repertoire.

Identity Construction and the Role of the Good Parent

There is a growing literature that explores wider systemic influences on people and their health and behaviour, but the dominant discourses remain centred around individual or family accountability. Throughout this chapter, we use several interrelated terms, for clarity the ways in which we use these terms are, parents are *responsible*, but when child does something that is deemed to be socially inappropriate, parents become *accountable*, which then justifies the social action of *blame*.

There is a strong social ideology of what it means to be a 'good parent', with parents being treated as responsible for their child's behaviour (Liahaugen Flensburg et al., 2022). This model of 'parental determinism' purports that a child's future is determined by their parent's abilities (Lind et al., 2016). The action and choices that parents make are typically used as a reference point to account for their children's social problems, such as school failure, drug problems, or criminal activity (Barker & Hunt, 2004). Although parental determinism relates to both mothers and fathers, it has been suggested that parenting practices continue to be gendered and mothers retain greater levels of involvement in child rearing (Fox, 2009). Social expectations about the role of women are influenced by cultural expectations and specifically what it means to be a 'good mother' (Collett, 2005). Cultural ideals of motherhood, therefore, affect not only how society perceives them, but also how they perceive themselves (Tabatabai, 2020).

It is fairly common when engaging with professionals working with families, for parents to feel that their parenting skills are being assessed (as often they in fact are). Against this backdrop of explicit or implicit evaluation, parents may seek to pro-actively demonstrate to professionals working with them, that they ought to be assessed as 'good' parents. The following two extracts from family therapy are examples of this. In the first extract, the father initiates a self-evaluation about himself and his partner about trying to be 'good parents'. In the second extract, the father evaluates his partner as 'good as a parent'. It is normal for people to compare and judge their parenting skills against the prevailing social norms about what constitutes a good parent (taken from O'Reilly & Lester, 2016, p. 499).

Niles family

```
Dad:   ↑Oh well >I mean< we try t' be good parents don't we >I
       mean< (1.2) I know he's not genetically mine but 'e gets
       (.) >I mean< I treat 'im like me own (.) >you know what
       I mean< he doesn't go without
FT:    You've been around for a long time Alex
```

Clamp family

```
FT:    Actually, Dan if I were t' ask Joanne where she rates
       herself as a parent (.) where do you think she would
       put herself
       (2.0)
Dad:   She's good as a parent
```

For parents who encounter criticisms for failure to meet societal expectations, they can experience significant stigmatisation and discrimination which can become internalised as parents worry about what others may think (Wilkens & Foote, 2019). Concerns about how they are perceived by others can cause parents to worry about their own parenting competencies, meaning that they, as parents of children who deviate from social norms can be labelled by society and themselves as a 'bad parent' (Trigueros et al., 2022). The very categories of 'good' and 'bad' are moral constructs, and therefore when a parent is labelled as a bad parent, it is intrinsically a moral judgment that has been passed on them. There is considerable evidence that children with mental health needs are often stigmatised, and by association, parents and family members are affected by what Goffman referred to as 'courtesy stigma' (Goffman, 1963).

> **Courtesy Stigma**
> The prejudice and discrimination that a stigmatised person encounters are also experienced by their family members and others close to them.

When working with families, it is important that practitioners are mindful of this potential for courtesy stigma and how family members might be experiencing discrimination by association (see also Chap. 1 for discussion). For example, research shows that those experiencing courtesy stigma have a greater likelihood of increased emotional distress and social isolation (Green, 2001). Notably, this stigmatisation may come from within the extended family (Moses, 2010), some of whom may be present in the institutional interaction. It is therefore important to recognise that courtesy stigma is not the only challenge for families, as there are many kinds of stigma that might be encountered, and we outline these in Table 8.1.

For a family seeking help, they may have already encountered 'experienced stigma' prior to their referral both directly and via association, that is, 'courtesy stigma'. In accessing support, they may also have experienced 'treatment stigma' from others and additionally may expect a degree of stigmatisation from practitioners they are seeking help from, that is, 'anticipated stigma'. Therefore, as family practitioners working in the context of mental health, it may be helpful to bear in mind these psychological barriers to accessing services and the vulnerabilities that families

Table 8.1 Different kinds of stigma (Clement et al., 2015)

Stigma type	Description
Experienced stigma	Direct experience of stigmatisation for being deviant from social norms
Perceived stigma	Belief of experiencing stigmatisation
Stigma endorsement	Agreement with stigmatising perceptions of others
Anticipated stigma	The expectation of being treated unfairly due to stigma
Internalised stigma	Acceptance of others' prejudice and stigmatisation, and a belief that this is warranted
Treatment stigma	A stigma associated with seeking help or treatment

face in relation to their expectations of social views of bad parenting. Additionally, and more problematically, family members may also be experiencing 'internalised stigma', where they have actually taken on negative self-perceptions and may blame themselves for their child's difficulties.

Parent Blaming

The idea of positioning parents, particularly mothers, as blameworthy for their child's mental health and behaviour has a long history. In modern European history, psychoanalysis was the dominant practice for managing mental health and was highly influential at the turn of the twenty-first century (Porter, 1997). With this theorising, there was an emphasis on the individual, and mothers were spotlighted as being the most prominent figure in the child's development (Lafrance & McKenzie-Mohr, 2013). It was during 1935 that tensions started to emerge with the publication of the first child psychiatry textbook by Leo Kanner (Karim, 2015) bringing the idea that child mental health could be medicalised, and the post-second world war challenges with the rise of attachment theories (Bone & Marchant, 2016). This was politically useful to use the research on attachment to propagate the idea that women who had been out at work during the war, should return to homes to look after their children. Shortly after, with concern about growing divorce rates came pressure on families to take responsibility for increases in what was positioned as juvenile delinquency, which was a precursor to family therapy (Dallos & Draper, 2010). We acknowledge that this is an extreme simplification, but for the purposes of introducing this chapter, we intend to demonstrate the socio-political influences that have shaped the ways that normality and deviance are constructed and the ways in which mental health services have adapted.

The legacy of those early conceptual frameworks about pathology being individualised and accountability for children's deviance being positioned within the family system is still evident today. Even in a modern society where gender equality is advocated, mothers are still positioned a primarily responsibility for the wellbeing of children (Jackson & Mannix, 2004), with a common expectation that the mother will put her child's needs before their own (Lind et al., 2016). Although fathers are becoming more visible, it is still mothers who typically take on much of the caring labour (Silverman, 2012). Thus, when children experience mental health difficulties, it is still culturally likely to blame the mother (Jackson, 2018), and mothers are often aware of this stigmatising practice, which can influence their help-seeking behaviour and service engagement (Jackson & Mannix, 2004).

> Parents who anticipate blame and stigma for their children's mental or behavioural health difficulties, may be reluctant to seek professional support. It is therefore important for practitioners to understand the reasons for this barrier to help-seeking and consider ways to make services more accessible.

Indeed, research has highlighted that some mothers of children with mental health conditions had experienced negative comments and even felt that clinical practitioners had treated them negatively due to the child's difficulty (Blum, 2007). Thus, in clinical settings, it is common for parents to try to discursively construct themselves as good parents (O'Reilly & Kiyimba, 2021), potentially due to their perception that they are being scrutinised by the clinical practitioners (Todd & Jones, 2003).

In addition to feeling stigmatised for being the parent of a child with a mental health difficulty or diagnosis, parents also face stigma when they have children who are struggling with addiction. As an example of this, a recent survey of 728 persons with a family member with addiction in New Zealand, reported that 45% felt embarrassed, 54% felt guilty, and 47% reported shame (Kiyimba & Scarlett, 2021). The authors of that study found that these are emotions that can inhibit help-seeking and accessing sources of support. In addition to feelings of guilt and shame, family members can also experience anxiety and depressive symptoms arising from the social judgements (Trigueros et al., 2022). These feelings of shame also extend to children and young people too as many tend to turn to peers for support rather than practitioners because of the stigma (Brophy & Holmstrom, 2006), and the feelings of embarrassment become a central barrier to their help seeking (Chandra & Minkovitz, 2006). We invite you to reflect on this challenge of blame and shame, by addressing the activity in Box 8.2.

Box 8.2 Reflective Activity: Overcoming Barriers to Help-Seeking

Reflective activity
  Overcoming barriers
  Although it is the child in the family identified as having the mental health condition, it is the parents who are the gatekeepers to access support for the child and there may be two significant barriers—one is their own challenges that arise from experiencing judgment and stigmatisation, and the other relates to fears of shame and blame from those they may be approaching for help.

- How can we as practitioners overcome these two barriers and facilitate family engagement with services?

Managing Responsibility and Blame

A well-established understanding of how children develop is the debate regarding biological causes (nature) combined with the influence of the environment (nurture). With regards to parents, they contribute both to the child's profile genetically and biologically, but also environmentally in terms of modelling learned behaviour. Whilst nature and nurture used to be positioned as binary concepts, an either/or causal explanation, it is now much more widely accepted that a child's development is influenced by a complex interplay of both. Nonetheless, in our data, we can see that parents draw upon this discursive repertoire of nature versus nurture as an explanatory resource for their child's problems.

In relation to the avoidance of blame, parents may explain their child's difficulties in terms of biological or genetic causes rather than environmental ones, thus working to absolve themselves from a blame position of poor parenting and mitigate any potential idea implication of them being poor parents. Thus, by constructing the child's behaviour and emotional challenges as related to an underlying health condition, and one that has a scientific or genetic foundation, parents can medicalise their child and move away from any potential consideration that this may be due to inappropriate nurturing and a lack of parental skills (O'Reilly & Kiyimba, 2021). The appeal to a scientific/biological discourse is one way of rhetorically managing their role in the child's health and absolving themselves of blame for their child's difficulties. A good example of this can be seen in the following extract where the parents are discussing their 16-year-old son who has been displaying inappropriate sexual behaviour toward his younger brother and others (taken from O'Reilly, 2014, p. 169).

Webber family

```
FT:     >I wuz gonna ask< (.) >you know< what kind of
        explanation::ns you have, fo::r (.) >you know< why it
        is that 'e's (.) he's ↑started doin' (.) <the:se things>
Mum:    <I don't know> (.) I ↑say it t' scho:ol (.) and >you
        know< there's this theory is it in the g::enes
```

LaFrance and McKenzie-Mohr (2013) suggest that drawing upon a biological explanatory framework is a way that people can manage and defend the way that others perceive their identity. In other words, a genetic account for a child's problem behaviour is proposed by the mother as preferred to the alternative. In the extract of data presented, the child's mother does two things. First, she positions the problem behaviour as '*in the genes*' and second, argues that the 'nature' explanation is one that was provided by an expert other, that is, the school. By reporting the expert opinion of another to support her own case, the mother adds weight to her proposal (see O'Reilly et al., 2023). In this way, a biological discursive construction of the child's mental health difficulties functions to absolve her from any potential assignation of blame for her inappropriate or deficient parenting skills as being the reason for the child's problem behaviour (Singh, 2002). We provide a second example of how parents draw on a discourse of a malfunction of the child's brain as an explanation, for their 14-year-old son's regular violent outbursts (as taken from O'Reilly, 2014, p. 169).

Niles family

```
Dad:      It's (.) as if he's got 'e's got a little tiny
          >microchip< in 'is brain an' 'e's sayin' (.) every
          now and again 'e just goes flip
FT:       ↓Right
Dad:      switches off and he lo:ses it
FT:       So. (.) the::re's an idea that it's, inherited o::r
          ↑possibly somethin' >t' do< with >I dunno<
Mum:      >His dad<
FT:       chemistry of (.) Steve's ↑bra:in
```

Here, the stepfather uses a lay metaphor to provide a biological aetiology of the child's mental health difficulty as internal, physiological, and pre-determined. By positioning the behaviour as stemming from a pre-existing biological irregularity, the stepfather constructs his parenting as responsive to, rather than causal of, the child's behaviour. The family therapist further clarifies that what the stepfather is suggesting is that the predisposition is 'inherited'. The risk of using a concept like 'inherited' is that there is a subtle suggestion that indirectly parents carry some responsibility. However, this is mitigated by the mother as she quickly interjects that any inherited behaviour is due to the biological, non-present father, not the stepfather who is present. A key aspect of identity construction that is at stake in this conversation relates to moral judgements. Social norms are inevitably interconnected with moral evaluations, and in an interaction like this, each of the parties involved is normatively involved in the process of attributing moral categories to people based on observed or reported behaviour (Roca-Cuberes, 2008).

Virtue Signalling and Identifying as a Good Parent

As discussed in the previous section, one of the ways of managing potential accountability and blame for the child's behaviour was to position it as biologically determined. By negotiating the child's difficulties as medical, parents negate other potential ascriptions that might imply the child's difficulties are because of their parenting practices. Another way that parents manage their parenting identity is to position themselves as virtuous. This is often done using examples of good parenting actions. The concept of virtue signalling is defined as deliberate statements constructed to highlight the virtuous or positive qualities of the speaker (Wallace et al., 2020).

> Virtue signalling can function to mitigate any possible perception that deficits in their parenting are the reasons for the child's difficulties.

The function of virtue signalling is to convince others of their moral respectability (Tosi & Warmke, 2016). What is often at stake for parents as they come into contact with professional services is that the practitioners working with them may attribute the child's difficulties to poor parenting. One way to guard against this judgement is for parents to find ways to present themselves as good parents, that is, stake inoculation. We present two examples from the mental health assessment data of parents 'doing a good parent identity' (taken from O'Reilly & Kiyimba, 2021, p. 6 of online version).

Family 11

```
Mum     [no he has ne]ver ↓crossed his the road on 'is own ↓you
        know I am [alw]ays with him
```

In this example, the mother describes her caution in keeping the child safe. Her use of the words 'never' and 'always' emphasise the point she is making that she takes her role as mother seriously and always looks after her child's best interests. These concepts are referred to as extreme case formulations (Pomerantz, 1986). In the following extract, a good parent identity is portrayed using the example of ensuring the child is adequately nourished despite the child's food refusal (taken from O'Reilly & Kiyimba, 2021, p. 6 of online version).

Family 26

```
Clin Psy    and if 'e is (.) if 'e won't eat somethin' how what
            would your re↓sponse to that?
Mum         I've always got a s[oup] in
Clin Psy                       [be]
Mum         (0.43)
            an:d soup is the standby really and [an']
Gran                                             [soup]
            an' cereal
Mum         soup and cereal yeah but most of the time he has:
            (I know) because I know what he likes and what he'll
            eat (0.57) and I'd rather him eat
```

In orienting to the child's food refusal, the clinical psychologist enquires of the mother how she manages the situation. The implication is that the question seeks clarification about the adequacy of her parental skills. In response, the mother acknowledges that a diet of soup is not ideal, but that she 'always' has some in the house as a 'standby'. By referring to this as a 'standby' indicates that this option is not her preferred choice, but her good parent identity is held intact by her diligence to ensure the child has something to eat.

Importantly, the efficacy of this strategy to present examples of good parenting actions relies on shared social norms of the kinds of behaviours that are expected of good parents. In the case of crossing the road and eating food, the virtue signalling of the mother in each case was successful because of these shared understandings. However, the following two extracts are examples of parents attempting to do virtue signalling through using examples of what they consider to be good parenting but fall short of wider societal social norms (taken from O'Reilly & Lester, 2016, p. 502).

Clamp family

```
Dad:      but we fini shed the course >what we did< on parenting
          but that was good (.) because we did lea:rn a lot on
          that it didn't help to smack children and
          ↑whatever ↓yeah
FT:       Yeah
Dad:      And we didn't we 'aven't smacked 'em for a long long
          time now >not unless< they've been really
          rea::lly bad
FT:       Hu::m
```

Clearly, a previous family professional had encouraged this couple to attend a parenting course to support their parenting skills, which the father refers to. In mentioning that they learned not to smack their children in this parenting course, the father reports that they have not used this punishment technique for a *'long long time'*. Ostensibly, this virtue signalling is effective in displaying improvement in their parenting skills. However, he adds the caveat *'unless they've been really really bad'*. In so doing, he undermines his presentation of self as a good parent because he potentially raises the question mark in the family therapist's mind about whether the children may at times be at risk (something we discuss in more detail in the next chapter).

When working with families, particularly in relation to child protection, there is a great deal at stake. Ultimately, there is the potential that the child may be removed from families if the practitioner believes that the child is at risk. Our data demonstrate that parents work hard to present themselves in a positive light, but may have a distorted view on what constitutes safe and responsible care of their children. Practitioners reading this book are likely aware of the need to gather information from a range of sources, as well as evaluating the parental accounts to make an informed decision about requirements for additional professional services. In conducting this professional role with families, there is a difference between judgement and evaluation. Judgement is a potentially negative view of families, whereas evaluation is a sober professional assessment.

Final Thoughts

Throughout this chapter, we have used the language of shame and blame to discuss the responsibility of parents in their children's mental health and wellbeing. This terminology is a colloquial way of engaging with the topic and is familiar in everyday encounters that families may experience. Within wider society, notions of parental responsibility and therefore accountability permeate. As practitioners working with families, it is helpful to be aware of these wider social narratives and, at the same time, be cautious about reproducing them within the institutional setting. While there may be helpful guidance that parents can be informed about to enhance their capacity to parent their children successfully, we suggest that recommendations for such interventions come from a place of professional integrity rather than negative judgements or stigmatisation. In Box 8.3, Erin O'Neill talks about the guilt, stigma, and shame felt by parents of adult children struggling with addiction.

To close our chapter, we summarise the key messages from that we feel are important for you in Box 8.4.

> **Box 8.3 Practitioner Voice, Erin O'Neill**
>
> Practitioner voices
> Erin O'Neill
> Support network lead
>
>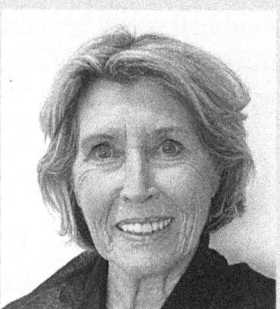
>
> Erin O'Neill understands the effects of addiction on family members: and was compelled to start Brave Hearts NZ—Manawa Kaha Aotearoa—a support network for whānau (the Māori word for extended family) and friends with a loved one in addiction. She felt families needed more peer support, education, and advocacy during this difficult time. Erin's tenacity has provided many with the help they've needed to get their family members into recovery and to move towards the ultimate goal of living addiction free.
>
> PLEASE DON'T JUDGE ME
>
> In the context of addiction, the family is an important institution. While it is the individual who has the issues, it is the whole network around them that needs the support for it to be a successful outcome for future generations. Families, therefore, are really asking themselves:
>
> - "Is there something wrong with me?"
> - "What did I do wrong in parenting the child?"
> - "Where did I go wrong with consequences in adolescent years?"
> - "Was I loving enough in my relationship with my partner, child, sibling?"
>
> How can I support and love an addict—someone who is terrorising me, often a criminal, and being a drain on rather than contributing to society?
>
> By showing that we are 'holding up really well', 'being a good member of society', this allows us to keep functioning but is really another layer of complexity thrown on top of what is already unbearable.
>
> *(continued)*

Box 8.3 (continued)

Specialist help is often seen as patronising, so families present as being there to obtain help for the addict—nothing wrong with me—no stigma attached. Professionals who work with families need to be aware that we become so overburdened by what we can't talk about—feelings of guilt, feeling of being ostracised in society, being seen as weak or frail.

We are too scared of judgement to show our vulnerability. We need to know that you can break down these barriers and allow us to talk frankly and openly without fear of how the rest of the world sees us. Listening, understanding without pre-conceived judgement. These are important areas of reflection for the practitioner working with families.

Organisations are starting to employ people with lived experience as they recognise the importance of involving experts by experience. This peer support is invaluable in the sector—like helping with total empathy—and so important, to receive the essential *element* of Hope that comes from an individual with a successful outcome.

Organisations must have a responsibility to mitigate stigma in the delivery of their service. More awareness of how to do this would ensure earlier help seeking and ultimately save time and money. Continuous development and learning from each other. Identify what is working well. Those who have the essential tools to help them cope find this unbearable time is shortened, thereby ensuring that the effects on both the family and the addict are not as severe.

Box 8.4 Key Points

- Wider negative societal discourses of parenting may leak into professional mental health conversations.
- Parents have a stake and interest in presenting themselves in a positive way within those interactions.
- Anticipation of being blamed for the child's difficulties, and the potential for stigma, may inhibit help-seeking.
- Family practitioners benefit from being aware of these issues around blame and responsibility, to be proactive in avoiding re-stigmatisation in institutional settings.

References

Barker, J., & Hunt, G. (2004). Representations of family: A review of the alcohol and drug literature. *International Journal of Drug Policy, 15*(5–6), 347–356.

Blum, L. (2007). Mother-blame in the Prozac nation: Raising kids with invisible disabilities. *Gender and Society, 21*(2), 202–226.

Bone, C., & Marchant, N. (2016). A critical discursive perspective on psychiatric hospitals. In *The Palgrave handbook of adult mental health* (pp. 459–477). Palgrave Macmillan.

Brophy, M., & Holmstrom, R. (2006). *Truth hurts: Report of the National Inquiry into self-harm among young people: Fact or fiction?* Mental Health Foundation.

Chandra, A., & Minkovitz, C. (2006). Stigma starts early: Gender differences in teen willingness to use mental health services. *Journal of Adolescent Health, 38*, 754.e1–754.e8.

Clement, S., Schauman, O., Graham, T., & Maggioni, F. (2015). What is the impact of mental health-related stigma on help-seeking? A systematic review of quantitative and qualitative studies. *Psychological Medicine, 45*(1), 11–27.

Collett, J. (2005). What kind of mother am I? Impression management and the social construction of motherhood. *Symbolic Interaction, 28*(3), 327–347.

Dallos, R., & Draper, R. (2010). *An introduction to family therapy: Systemic theory and practice* (3rd ed.). Open University Press.

Fox, B. (2009). *When couples become parents: The creation of gender in the transition to parenthood.* University of Toronto Press.

Goffman, E. (1963). *Stigma: Notes on the management of a spoiled identity.* Prentice Hall.

Green, S. (2001). Oh, those therapists will become your best friends: Maternal satisfaction with clinics providing physical, occupational and speech therapy services to children with disabilities. *Sociology of Health and Illness, 23*, 798–828.

Jackson, I. (2018). What impact does an adult substance user have on mothers, and how do they make sense of their experience? *Universal Journal of Psychology, 6*(1), 19–28.

Jackson, D., & Mannix, J. (2004). Giving voice to the burden of blame: A feminist study of mothers' experiences of mother blaming. *International Journal of Nursing Practice, 10*, 150–158.

Karim, K. (2015). The value of conversation analysis: A child psychiatrist's perspective. In M. O'Reilly & J. N. Lester (Eds.), *The Palgrave handbook of child mental health: Discourse and conversation studies* (pp. 25–41). Palgrave Macmillan.

Kiyimba, N., & Scarlett, E. (2021). The cost of addiction for families and whānau: A collaborative research project between brave hearts and Bethlehem Tertiary Institute, AFINet 2021 conference, September, UK.

Lafrance, M., & McKenzie-Mohr, S. (2013). The DSM and its lure of legitimacy. *Feminism and Psychology, 23*(1), 119–140.

Liahaugen Flensburg, O., Johnson, B., Nordgren, J., Richert, T., & Svensson, B. (2022). "Something wasn't right"—parents of children with drug problems looking back at how the troubles first began. *Drugs: Education, Prevention and Policy, 29*(3), 255–264.

Lind, A., Westerling, A., Sparrman, A., & Dannesboe, K. (2016). Introduction: Doing good parenthood. In A. Sparrman, A. Westerling, J. Lind, & K. Dannesboe (Eds.), *Doing good parenthood* (pp. 1–16). Palgrave Macmillan Studies in Family and Intimate Life.

Moses, T. (2010). Exploring parents' self-blame in relation to adolescents' mental disorders. *Family Relations, 59*(2), 103–120.

O'Reilly, M. (2014). Blame and accountability in family therapy: Making sense of therapeutic spaces discursively. [Special issue]. *Qualitative Psychology, 1*(2), 163–177.

O'Reilly, M., & Kiyimba, K. (2021). Responsibility inoculation: Constructing 'good parent' accounts when accessing child mental health services. *Human Systems: Therapy, Culture & Attachment, 1*(1), 52–69.

O'Reilly, M., Kiyimba, N., Lee, V., & Hutchby, I. (2023). Give my child a label: Strategies of epistemic corroboration in case-building within child mental health assessments. *Sociology, 1*, 20.

O'Reilly, M., & Lester, J. N. (2016). Building a case for good parenting in a family therapy systemic environment: Resisting blame and accounting for children's behaviour. *Journal of Family Therapy, 38*(4), 491–511.

Pomerantz, A. (1986). Extreme case formulations: A way of legitimizing claims. *Human Studies, 9*(2–3), 219–229.

Porter, R. (1997). *The greatest benefit to mankind: A medical history of humanity from antiquity to the present*. Harper Collins Publishers.

Roca-Cuberes, C. (2008). Membership categorization and professional insanity ascription. *Discourse Studies, 10*(4), 543–570.

Silverman, C. (2012). *Understanding autism: Parents, doctors, and the history of a disorder*. Princeton University Press.

Singh, I. (2002). Bad boys, good mothers, and the "miracle" of Ritalin. *Science in Context, 15*(4), 577–603.

Tabatabai, A. (2020). Mother of a person: Neoliberalism and narratives of parenting children with disabilities. *Disability & Society, 35*(1), 111–131.

Todd, S., & Jones, S. (2003). 'Mum's the word!': Maternal accounts of dealings with the professional world. *Journal of Applied Research in Intellectual Disabilities, 16*, 229–244.

Tomm, K., George, S. S., Wulff, D., Strong, T., & (Eds.). (2014). *Patterns in interpersonal interactions: Inviting relational understandings for therapeutic change*. Routledge.

Tosi, J., & Warmke, B. (2016). Moral grandstanding. *Philosophy & Public Affairs, 44*(3), 197–217.

Trigueros, R., Navarro, N., Mercader, I., Aguilar-Parra, J. M., Lopez-Liria, R., & Rocamora-Pérez, P. (2022). Self-stigma, mental health, and healthy habits in parent of children with severe mental disorder. *Psychology Research and Behavior Management, 15*, 227.

Wallace, E., Buil, I., & De Chernatony, L. (2020). 'Consuming good' on social media: What can conspicuous virtue signalling on Facebook tell us about prosocial and unethical intentions? *Journal of Business Ethics, 162*(3), 577–592.

Wilkens, C., & Foote, J. (2019). "Bad Parents," "Codependents," and other stigmatizing myths about substance use disorder in the family. In J. Avery & J. Avery (Eds.), *The stigma of addiction* (pp. 33–53). Springer.

9

How to Talk About Risk

Learning Objectives

- Recognise the importance of asking families about risk
- Critically assess different strategies for asking about risk
- Evaluate when confidentiality might be breached
- Identify methods of self-care

Introduction

Risk is a ubiquitous concept and one that has multiple meanings in relation to working with children and families. In simplistic terms, the Oxford English Dictionary (2018, n.p.) defines risk in the following way:

Risk
A situation involving exposure to danger.

In the context of families, there is an onus on most professionals to engage in formal or informal risk assessment when working with families, and there is a duty of care to take steps to protect family members or members of the public who may potentially be at risk from harm (or danger). Risk can take different forms and each of these needs to be considered:

- Risk of harm to self.
- Risk of harm to others.
- Risk of harm from others.

Risk to self includes challenges like self-harm, suicidal ideation, but also risk-taking behaviours like promiscuity, excessive alcohol use, dangerous driving, and conversely neglect behaviour such as failing to adhere to medication, not attending hospital appointments, and neglecting self-care.

Risk to others includes being a perpetrator of aggressive behaviour, carrying a weapon, researching violent acts on the internet, cyberbullying, gang culture, and general antisocial behaviour but also intimate partner violence.

Risk from others includes being a victim of childhood sexual abuse, emotional abuse, physical abuse, bullying, grooming, trolling, but also intimate partner violence.

In discussions of risk, it is also necessary to consider what is meant by harm. There are different types of harm that need to be accounted for in the risk assessment and practitioners should consider the moral, legal, physical, emotional, sexual, and psychological aspects of harm. These can be thought of as along three dimensions:

1. The type of harm—such as physical, psychological, and social harm.
2. The severity of the harm—in terms of the impact it has on the individual and others.
3. The longevity of the harm—how long the impact influences the individual (Source: Livingstone, 2013).

> Physical harm refers to injury or damage to the body, psychological harm refers to mental harm from others, such as emotional invalidation or gas-lighting, as well as indirect consequences such as anxiety, depression, or flashbacks. Social harm refers to damage to relationships either within the family, or between friends or colleagues, or even wider reputational social harm.

When having conversations with families, professionals need to be aware of all the different potential aspects of risk and types of harm, as well as the potential overlap between them.

In accounting for risk-taking behaviour of the family members, developmental age and maturity are factors to consider. Younger children are developing their ability to regulate emotion and the language required to articulate their feelings (Zeman et al., 2006). At different life stages, peer influence rather than parental influence becomes more prominent. Adolescents are more likely to be fiercely loyal to their peers (Blakemore, 2018), sometimes to their detriment. Adolescents are at a developmental period during puberty where prefrontal cortex development means they have less impulse control and are more likely to engage in risk-taking behaviour (Steinberg, 2010). Older adults, especially those with some forms of dementia (frontotemporal dementia) also may be at greater risk of inappropriate social behaviour and neglecting their self-care (Plaisted & Sahakian, 1997).

Furthermore, there may be ambiguity as to whether the child or adult is the victim or perpetrator. Children witnessing violence between different members of the family would also be considered to be harm to the child. A child or adult can both be a perpetrator and victim. Thus, in working with the family, it is important to be cognisant of the intersections and overlapping nature of risk. Three examples are provided below:

- Because the child's father is in prison, a child may be a victim of cyberbullying from peers and uses self-harming to manage the emotional distress.
- A mother who is a victim of intimate partner violence may in turn physically or emotionally abuse her children.
- An older sibling who has been sexually abused by an uncle may engage in inappropriate sexual behaviour towards a younger sibling.

> A family member may be both a victim and perpetrator – they are thus a risk to others and from others.

While there are a range of possible risk situations in the three domains, for the purpose of clarity in this chapter, we focus on three main areas: (1) communicating about risk of self-harm and suicidal ideation; (2) questions about intimate partner/domestic violence; and (3) engaging in dialogue about behaviours that might potentially put others at risk.

How to Have a Conversation About Risk

Practitioners may be reluctant to engage in conversations about risk, due to concerns of making the situation worse (Bajaj et al., 2008) or a lack of confidence in how to do so, or concerns about time constraints to fully explore the issue. Notably, evidence shows that talking about suicide and self-harm does not directly increase or cause those behaviours (Dazzi et al., 2014) and may instead reduce suicidality (Aseltine et al., 2007). It is often the case that practitioners working with families may be the first to identify possible risk of harm to self or to or from others, amongst family members. Indeed, professional ethics may dictate that it is a professional responsibility to be aware of these possibilities.

We recommend readers to remind themselves of the professional obligations and ethical context of your own particular professional guidelines with regard to risk identification and management before reading further. Most professions have a professional body to which you will have membership or affiliation, and this professional body will typically publish ethical requirements for that profession. Our examples that follow demonstrate different ways to ask family members about possible risk, but do not address how that risk is managed once it has been disclosed. It is very likely that the organisation that you work for will have a set of guidelines that clearly outline what the steps and processes are in managing risk once it has been disclosed.

> One of the first priorities in any new professional context is to locate and familiarize yourself with the risk management policies. It is essential that when a family member discloses an area of risk, that you are aware of what the appropriate course of action is.

Using data examples, we focus on the three main domains of harm; harm to self, harm to others and harm from others to contextualise and conceptualise communication strategies for engaging families in conversations about risk.

Harm to Self

> **Harm to Self**
> Traditionally, harm to self refers to physical acts of deliberate self-injury. More recently, a broader definition includes different ways that people cause harm to themselves psychologically, including aliases on online platforms to verbalise negative criticisms about themselves.

When working with families, it is important to address potential risk of harm to self, such as deliberate actions to cause physical harm and/or suicidal thoughts or plans. Evidence shows that globally more than 800,000 people die by suicide annually (World Health Organization [WHO], 2019), and it is the second leading cause of death in 15–19-year-olds (WHO, 2014). In England and Wales, suicide is the leading cause of death for 5–19-year-olds (Office for National Statistics, 2016). These shocking statistics demonstrate that it is a very real problem and therefore it is important that we find ways to talk openly about suicide and self-harm with children as well as adults. It is even more important to have explicit conversations if any of the following risk factors are identified within the family:

- Mental health conditions and/or history of self-harm.
- Alcohol or substance misuse.
- Physical illness (particularly chronic disability).
- Economic challenges such as job loss, poverty, or debt.
- Family difficulties.
- Adverse Childhood Experiences (ACEs).
- Bereavement by suicide or previous suicide attempt.
- Certain vulnerabilities, including LGBQT+, asylum-seeking status, incarceration, or risk occupations.
  (Source: Klonsky et al., 2017; Piotrowski & Hartmann, 2019)

Recent evidence suggests that self-harm in children has increased in prevalence (NHS Digital, 2019). Females between 10 and 14 years are particularly at risk (Griffin et al., 2018) and even children as young as seven years are engaging in behaviours that cause physical harm to themselves and presenting to hospital with their injuries (Barrocas et al., 2012). Notably, the prevalence rates may be even higher as self-harm in children is underreported (Hawton et al., 2012) due to their anxiety about disclosure (Bostik & Everall, 2006). As practitioners, therefore, it is important to remember to ask about risk of harm to self and not assume that a child will volunteer to self-disclose, and to ask even young children this question. The following extract (that we referred to in chapter four), demonstrates the importance of this as the child is only nine years old and discloses suicidal intention (taken from Kiyimba & O'Reilly, 2018, p. 152).

Family 6   (Prac = Psychiatrist)

```
Prac    so when you ↓said that you were going to take a ↓knife
        to yourself
        (0.99)
Prac    yeah?
        (1.15)
Prac    what were you ↓hoping would happen?
Child   erm (2.45) f::or me to ↓actually kill my↓self
```

As discussed earlier in the book, if the child has previously disclosed self-harm activity, the 'you said x' preface is a helpful way to reintroduce the topic and encourage elaboration. However, if a child does not volunteer a disclosure and the onus is on you as a practitioner to initiate the conversation. Indeed, this responsibility may be an integral aspect of your professional role. We suggest two ways to do this based on our analysis of practitioners asking about risk. These are, asking about risk incrementally or asking about risk in a way that normalises the question.

Incremental

If a child has not given any indication of self-harm behaviour, it might feel a bit difficult to suddenly ask direct risk question. However, failure to ask may be contravening the professional ethics of your role in working with families, which is often to prioritise risk assessment as part of the intervention. We found that building up to a direct question can make this process easier for the practitioner and the child and is likely to be more successful. An incremental way of asking questions about risk is to take a step-by-step approach, gradually building from questions about emotions and emotional regulation, and based on the answers working up to questions about suicidality. The following extract is taken from (O'Reilly et al., 2016, p. 483).

Family 18

```
Prac        Is there any other way you show your frustration
            (0.91) you said you hit
YP          Yeah I h[it doors] hit doors
Prac               [doors]
YP          there's a massive hole in my door
Prac        Yeah so you hit doors anything else?
YP          No
Prac        Or hurting yourself?
YP          Yeah
Prac        What d'you do?
YP          I slit my wrists once
((lines omitted))
Prac        Is there an intention to kill yourself?
YP          I (0.31) like (0.39) stupid things like taking loads
            of paracetamol or som'ing (0.78) somfing like that
Prac        Have you ever done that?
YP          Yeah
```

The way the practitioner creates an opportunity to start talking about risk is to initially ask about how the child exhibits his *'frustration'*. When he states that he *'hits doors'*, the open question *'anything else?'* allows for potential exploration of harm to self or others. The practitioner takes the opportunity, even after the child says no, to explicitly ask about harm to self *'or hurting yourself?'*. This proves to be a very important question, because when the child says yes and the practitioner asks how, the child discloses cutting his wrists.

> In this example, it is likely the child would not have disclosed if he had not been asked directly and the consequences might have been serious.

The practitioner could potentially have stopped at this point having identified information about self-harm from the child, however, the practitioner continues to directly ask about suicidal intention and finds out that the child has engaged in suicidal behaviour previously by taking *'loads of paracetamol'*. This extract demonstrates how a practitioner can incrementally lead up to direct questions about suicidal intention. It also shows that the practitioner must be bold enough to specifically use unambiguous language like *'hurting yourself'* and *'kill yourself'* to collect the relevant risk information.

Normalising

In situations where there seems to be no indication from the child, from their family or from the referral that there are any risks of harm to self, a normalising approach to asking may be the most appropriate. Normalising contextualises asking a risk question as merely a procedural requirement, and the question is not specific to the individual child but would be asked of all individuals attending the appointment. We provide an example of this (taken from O'Reilly et al., 2016, p. 484)

Family 21

```
Prac   This is a question we have to ask everybody an' I'm
       sure that you've been asked it before (1.38) when you
       feel (0.92) a bit frustrated or a bit sad (0.63) an' I
       know that you've punched walls before have you ever
       thought about (0.41) really hurting yourself
YP     No
```

> **Box 9.1 Reflective Activity on Questions About Risk**
>
> Reflective activity
>   Questions about risk
>   Thinking of these two types of risk questions and reflecting on the clients you work with, which of these questions might be most useful and when?
>
> - Have you ever used either of these questions?
> - How would you use a normalising question?
> - How do you feel about using an incremental approach to asking about risk?

The characteristics of a normalising approach to asking about risk are that it is presented as something that must be done and everybody who attends the service needs to be asked. This is demonstrated in the extract where the practitioner states *'this is a question we have to ask everybody'*. If you, as a practitioner feel concerned about how to ask about risk, this is a simple phrase that can be memorised and used in whatever context you are in. It can be followed up (as in this extract) with the question *'have you ever thought about really hurting yourself'*. We encourage you to attempt the reflective activity in Box 9.1.

Harm to Others

> **Harm to Others**
>
> Refers to physical, sexual, or psychological deliberate acts of harm to others in the family or wider social network. Neglect is also a form of harm to others.

In addition to assessing for risk of harm to self, assessing the risk of harm to others is another important consideration in many professional contexts working with families. Harm to others includes challenges such as intimate partner violence, child abuse, or violent/criminal behaviour in society. Harm to others also includes neglect. This may be particularly salient in relation to younger or older family members, or family members with additional needs that require help from others. Where family members have less capacity to look after themselves for various reasons and require the support of others, the very real risk of neglect may be present, and this is another form of harm to be aware of. Within a family context, there may be dynamics such that there is both harm from others and harm to others occurring. For example, in the context of intimate partner violence, one parent may be the perpetrator and the other the victim within the same family, and children who witness this intimate partner violence would also be classed as being harmed. All these things can be discussed within the family session with the practitioner. For the sake of simplicity, and to remain close to the data that we have collected, we discuss harm to others focusing on the child being a risk to other people within the family or outside of it and discuss issues like intimate partner violence and child abuse in relation to harm from others.

As we noted in our introduction, it is important to acknowledge there are different ways of defining harm, legally and morally. The notion of harm thus potentially includes a range of different types of offence (Baker, 2010). According to Her Majesty's Inspectorate of Probation (2008, p. 7), the purpose of assessing harm is to enable "*satisfactory clarification of the differences between the likelihood/probability of an event occurring and the impact/severity of the event*". This description captures the two main foci in relation to assessing the possibility of harm, which are probability and the impact. One of the measures to assess probability of harm occurring in the future is to consider historical acts of harm, their recency, frequency, and severity to predict the likelihood of future harm.

In the next two data extracts, the practitioner is engaging in a family therapy conversation about known historical harm perpetrated against one child in the family towards the sibling.

Webber family (taken from O'Reilly & Parker, 2014, p. 298)

```
Mother:   <he [the sibling] was touchin' our Stuart up> and
          >you know< when he's been doin' it 'cause he's got
          an erection all the while
FT:       Yeah
Mother:   and he's bloody embarrassin'
```

Here, the mother is describing to the family therapist the sexually inappropriate behaviour of one son towards another sibling, and her concerns about that. Thus, in terms of risk assessment knowledge about this recent risk activity is important in evaluating the likelihood of ongoing harm to Stuart, the younger sibling. Although the mother in this family highlights the conversation about this as being *'embarrassing'*, it is important for the practitioner to sensitively engage in finding out sufficient information to know whether a formal intervention is necessary to protect the younger siblings. Later in the session with the same family, based on the disclosures of the children's inappropriate sexual behaviour, the family therapist identifies the need to raise a safeguarding concern and involve social services.

> Conversations about risk and harm might be embarrassing, difficult or create additional workload, it is essential to prioritize the safety of all involved.

From Webber family—(previously unpublished data)

```
FT:    I mean without kind of raising your own anxieties
       what's kind of (name) (0.4) social services [doin'
Dad:                                                [They
       do nothin'
Mum:   They do nothin'
FT:    Are they are they aware of this latest incident?
Mum:   No
Dad:   No they're not aware of it 'cause (name) only comes in
       every now and then anyway
((Lines omitted))
FT:    I mean I guess there's a bit of me that thinks it's
       really important to hear about you know what's
       happening with Daniel (0.4) and and your thoughts on
       it (0.2) there's another bit of me that's kind of
       thinking (0.2) that actually performing oral sex on his
```

```
younger brother is quite serious (.) and do we need to
be telling social servic- I know they're already aware
of things in the past (0.6) and I'm not sure how they'd
react anyway 'cause I think (0.2) I think they are
clear that the two of you are working very hard
```

The social worker, is already involved with the family; however, the family therapist does not make any assumptions that she is aware of the most recent *'incident'*. The family therapist explicitly asks about this and finds out that social services are unaware of the current situation. The challenge for the therapist is to both fulfil his duty of care to protect the younger sibling from further harm and to hopefully maintain a positive therapeutic relationship with the parents. This can be seen in his validation of their efforts to *'work very hard'* in their parenting and his demonstration that he values their *'thoughts'* about what is happening. Simultaneously he manages to explain clearly to the parents that for the 16-year-old older brother to be *'actually performing oral sex on his younger brother is quite serious'*. Thus, the therapist manages to minimise the implied blame on their parenting ability while managing his duty of care to clearly explain the reasons for his need to involve social services. Ultimately, while the family therapist would have contacted social services about this safeguarding matter, he did so in a way that engaged the parents' acceptance and helped them to also see the seriousness of the situation.

While assessing for the risk of harm to others within the family and home environment is important, including direct harm and neglect, it is also necessary for practitioners to consider any potential for harm to others outside of the familial context. We provide two examples of this from the mental health assessment data now (the first is taken from O'Reilly & Kiyimba, 2019, n.p.).

Family 14

```
MHN      Have you ever been in trouble with the po↓lice
Child    [Ye:ah] ((laughs))
Mum      [yes]
MHN      °okay tell me a bit about that°
Child    I beat up someone (.) an' then
         (0.87)
         I [went]
MHN        [°(when) was] tha:t°
         (1.44)
         when [(was that)?]
Child         [this ↓wa:s]
Mum      in the summer
Child    um::: in the summer yeah =
MHN      this summer?
Child    ↑yeah
MHN      why did you beat them up?
Child    because like (.) they nearly got me battered
         (1.52)
         an:[d (   )]
MHN         [an' how ba]dly did you beat them ↓up
Child    Put 'em in hospital=
Mum      =This girl were bullying other ↓people: an' (name) just
         had just enough (of that)
```

An indirect way of introducing a conversation about risk of harm to others is demonstrated by the practitioner when she asks the child whether they have been in trouble with the police. Following an affirmative response, this provides a platform for the practitioner to explore more details about the offences. One of the key considerations in assessing for risk of potential harm to others in the future is establishing whether there has been actual harm to others historically, especially in the recent past. This is demonstrated in the extract when the practitioner asks, *'when was that?'* and for clarification about the recency of the behaviour, *'this summer?'* Another consideration in completing a risk assessment of this kind, is the severity of the historical incident of aggression, which is demonstrated when the practitioner asks, *'how badly did you beat them up?'* A final consideration demonstrated in this extract is the context of the historical incident of harm to others. Seeking this information establishes the context of the prior event. In this extract, the practitioner questions the reasons for the behaviour *'why did you beat them up?'*

By combining this information, the practitioner can make a judgement about the likelihood of future risk of harm to others, whether that risk might be restricted to certain contexts, and if it occurred, how severe the consequences might be. What is interesting about this example is that risk of harm to others is intrinsically connected to the potential of risk of harm from others. This can be seen in the collaborative rationale provided by the child and her mother that the child's actions were responsive to another child's initiation of aggression (bullying). Thus, the child reports *'they nearly got me battered'*, and the mother elucidates *'this girl were bullying other people'*. The following example (from previously unpublished data) demonstrates a similar complexity in the interrelationship between potential harm from and to others.

Family 8

```
Doctor     Coz your mum was ↓saying that you staying you stay
           (.) out ↓till quite late don't ↓you?
           (0.48) ((child nods head))
           An' what do you ↑do?
Child      ↓Play out
Doctor     ↑With
Child          (    )
Doctor     That's pretty ↓dangerous isn't it?
Child      Um
Doctor     ↓Are you scared?
Child      No
Doctor     ↓No
           (0.88)
           h[ow (full)]
Child        [I always] ↓carry ( ) and a screwdriver
           (around) with me
Doctor     Really?
```

For whatever reason, this child who is only 11 years old is having a conversation with the psychiatrist about 'playing out' late at night. The psychiatrist displays concern about the child's safety *'that's pretty dangerous'* and *'are you scared?'*. The child's disclosure of carrying the *'screwdriver'* is an indication of his perceived need to use a weapon to potentially defend himself. The complexity of this risk assessment therefore rests on establishing which of the two dimensions of risk is more problematic and likely; whether the child is more at risk of harm from others by being out late at night and/or whether he is a risk of harming others by using a screwdriver as a weapon or being arrested by the police for carrying a weapon.

Depending on the country and professional context, a mental health practitioner may have a duty of care to protect members of society from individuals who could pose a threat by taking further safeguarding actions. In other situations, such as in Canada for example, the mental health professional may be the one that continues to provide therapy and refers on to child protection officials if there is concern about violence or neglect. The child protection official then does the safety-associated work. Whether you are the practitioner responsible for the child protection aspect and/or the therapeutic side of supporting a family, establishing what the risk may be is an important step, so as to be clear about whether a referral is required. It is therefore important to ask appropriate questions to establish the severity of historical risk as an indicator of potential future risk.

Notably, within family systems, it is apparent that a risk of harm to others is often interconnected with an actual or potential risk of harm from others either within or outside the family. In our last example, there is an implicit question about what motivates a young child to risk being out at night rather than being at home, and whether the home environment poses greater risks, as well as the motivations for carrying the screwdriver. The challenge for practitioners in family conversations of this kind is that family members may be strongly motivated to protect their own interests. Thus, it is important to build therapeutic trust and alignment with each family member to foster an environment where asking these kind of questions might be more successful or productive.

Harm from Others

> **Harm from Others**
> Refers to negative physical, psychological, and sexual acts from others that may be deliberate, intentional, accidental, or consequential.

There are potentially various ways in which family members might be at risk of harm from others within or outside of the family. Two major areas of concern for practitioners are intimate partner violence (IPV) and child abuse in its various forms. Neglect is also another serious risk concern. In the UK, 7.3% of women (1.6 million) and 3.6% of men (757,000) had experienced domestic violence (now more commonly referred to as IPV), with women aged 16–19 years more likely to be victims than those over 25 years (Office for National Statistics, 2020). This is further complicated by the connection between children witnessing IPV and being physically abused (Kaufman & Henrich, 2000), with the likelihood of mothers in violent relationships being physically aggressive towards their children increasing (Lutenbacher et al., 2004). These statistics illustrate how important it is for practitioners to address risk of harm from others. Hornor (2005) provides a list of example questions that relate to assessing for risk of IPV and child abuse in the family home, which is reproduced in Box 9.2. The following reflective activity lists these prompt questions, and we invite you to consider which of these are useful in your professional context.

In addition to assessing for risk of IPV in relation to adult risk of harm from or to others, child witnesses of IPV within the family home also constitutes harm to the child. Therefore, when considering the impact of IPV, the risk of harm to the child should also be assessed. The following extract is an example of this.

```
Hand I um couldn't get breath and I um couldn't get breath and
my daughter of six years old was also there in my room, but
she's used to that.
```

(Taken from Dekel & Andipatin, 2016, n.p.)

> **Box 9.2 Reflective Activity on IPV and Child Abuse Questions (Hornor, 2005, p. 209)**
>
> Reflective activity
>   IPV and child abuse questions
>   *Questions to ask a parent*
>
> 1. Do you ever feel afraid in your home?
> 2. What happens when you and ___ (partner's name) argue?
> 3. Do arguments ever become physical? (i.e., hitting, kicking, pushing, throwing, or punching/breaking objects)
> 4. Have you ever been threatened with a weapon? (e.g., gun, knife, other)
> 5. Have you ever felt trapped or like a prisoner in your own home? Does your partner ever lock you in/out of the house or take your car keys?
> 6. Have your children ever seen or heard violence in the home?
> 7. Have the police ever been involved due to violence in your home?
> 8. Is the violence ever directed at the children? Does ___ (partner's name) ever hit, kick, push, or yell at your child when she/he is angry?
> 9. How do you and ___ (partner's name) discipline the children?
>
> *Questions to ask a child*
>
> 1. What happens when mommy and daddy (or appropriate partner names) argue/fight? Is there any hitting, pushing, and so on?
> 2. How do you feel when mommy and daddy (or appropriate partner names) fight?
> 3. What happens to you when you get in trouble?
> 4. If hitting or other physical forms of discipline occur, ask the following:
>   (a) What are you hit with?
>   (b) Where on your body?
>   (c) Does it ever leave a mark/bruise?
>   (d) Who hits/kicks you?
>   (e) How often does it happen?

Often people who are in situations where there is IPV and/or child abuse, it can become so 'normal' to them that they often do not perceive it as being abuse. As the example shows, the woman highlights how normative it is for her six-year-old daughter to witness violence in the family home, *'but she's used to that'*. Similarly, in our data, we observed instances where children were involved in episodes of violence in the home. In the following example, the father describes how his eldest son was punching the younger sibling, and he intervened to discipline the elder son by *'smacking'* his bum. The father presents his action as normative and proportional to the incident. However, it is likely to be perceived by others as constituting abuse because of the disclosure of using a *'belt'* to do so.

Clamp family (from O'Reilly, 2008, p. 284)

```
Dad:    >and h'e was bangin' 'is 'ead< (.) <against the wall>
        punching 'im in the face and everythin' (.) when I told
        'im to leave 'im alone, 'e told me ↑no
FT:     Hu::m
Dad     So (.) >I said< right >fair enough< (.) you've gone too
        far now (.) so I <took me belt off> and smacked 'is
        bum twice
FT:     Hu::m
Dad:    But (0.8) I bruised 'im (.) >he bruises easy
        anyway< er,
FT:     Hu::m
```

In relation to an assessment of risk of harm from others, the practitioner's duty of care is to ascertain the recency, frequency, and severity of the 'discipline' of the child to inform the formulation as to the likelihood of ongoing risk in the future. In this example, the father gives information about the recency of the event and provides a discourse of his construction of the severity of the event. The context to this disclosure is that a member of staff at the child's school had observed the bruises on the child's bottom and had reported it to social services. Thus, the father's version that the child bruises easily and that the punishment was appropriate and proportionate to the child's violent behaviour towards his brother constructs the act as reasonable and normal parental reaction.

> Bear in mind that the same member of the family might be a risk of harm to others as well as a risk of harm from others.

Our second example (and one that we included in an earlier chapter) is similar in the sense that the same father is disclosing another physical disciplinary action towards his eldest son.

Clamp family (From O'Reilly, 2008, p. 288)

```
Dad:      >you see< (0.4) with me punchin' 'im yesterd'y ↑yeah
          >I mean< .hh I do admit >I did punch 'im<
FT:       ↓Hu::m
Dad:      Yeah, >but< I didn't punch 'im >in the way to< (.)
          >you know w- I mean< I didn't <violent punch 'im>
FT:       ↓Right
Dad:      But (0.6) it it had to take that ↑punch
FT:       Right.
```

Again, while the father admits to a physical act of harm towards his son, he once more denies that it could be construed as an act of abuse or violence *'I didn't violent punch him'*. This shows that family members are not always subjectively very clear about what kinds of physical discipline would be regarded by wider society as abusive. Additionally, the father's argument consists of an account that appeals to the necessary and proportional nature of his response, *'it had to take that punch'*. In other words, the father argues that in order to maintain discipline of his son, it was necessary to punch him. We acknowledge both the fact that there are cultural differences in what is acceptable physical discipline, and also that what is appropriate is socially constructed and varies over time. However, within the context of our current societal rules, there are legal frameworks that dictate what constitutes abuse for the protection of the most vulnerable. Therefore, although the father in this example seems unaware that his actions are excessive and therefore inappropriate, it is the responsibility of the family practitioner to identify these extreme forms of discipline to ensure the children's safety.

The therapist's role, then, in these cases is to ascertain from the information presented the levels and severity of risk to take any immediate necessary action to involve social services, and once this is established, they can move forward to help the family find alternative ways to manage emotions and to communicate effectively without resorting to aggressive behaviour. Assessing risk of harm from others (and to others) is complicated for the practitioner. In our examples, we have shown the complexity of assessing risk of harm, by illustrating the fact that the younger brother is at risk from the older brother and the older brother is also at risk of harm from his father. Thus, the oldest son's behaviour constitutes a risk of harm *to* others, but he is simultaneously at risk of harm *from* his father. Our next example (which we used in chapter seven also) further illustrates the intricacies of assessing risk in family systems.

Clamp family (taken from O'Reilly & Parker, 2014, p. 294)

```
Dad:    She <turned round> and told my brother <in front of
        the three children> (.) <that 'e cannot 'ave anythin'
        t' do wiv ↑my children because 'e 'as sex with
        children>
FT:     ↓Right
```

Ostensibly, the immediate risk to the children is the possibility of sexual abuse from their uncle, who is already on the sex offender's register for sexual offences against a minor. A more subtle risk is the exposure of children to topics and language that are developmentally inappropriate. In this example, the father complains that the social worker '*she*' made explicit reference to his brother having '*sex with children*' whilst his children were present. On face value, this is an inappropriate form of action for the social worker to take. However, in reporting this misdemeanour to the therapist in the current interaction, the father repeats the same words again in front of his children who are present. Although we have not prioritised psychological harm in this section, this is nonetheless just as important for practitioners to assess for. Psychological harm refers to the damage done by words or actions that either undermine a person's sense of self-worth or expose them to information that could create anxiety, or fear, or as in this example, expose someone to information that is age-inappropriate.

Risk of Harm to Self, Others and from Others Online

When undertaking assessments of risk to self, to others and from others, it is important to be mindful that some of that ought to focus on how risk can be mediated through a digital environment. Notably, adolescents globally are highly engaged with digital devices (O'Reilly et al., 2021) at a developmental period that (as we noted earlier in the book) is associated with higher risk-taking (Steinberg, 2010), and therefore it is for practitioners to understand the intersection between risk and the internet. One recent taxonomy proposed was the four C's:

- Conduct—relates to children's behaviour online, for example, cyberbullying.
- Contact—relates to who they are communicating with online, for example, grooming.
- Content—relates to what they are reading/viewing online, for example, pornography.
- Contract—relates to seeing the child as a consumer, for example, inappropriate advertising. (Source: Livingstone & Stoilova, 2021)

In a similar way to assessing harm in person, the guidance on the risk of harm in a digital environment considers three dimensions:

1. The type of harm—such as physical, psychological, and social harm.
2. The severity of the harm—in terms of the impact it has on the individual.
3. The longevity of the harm—how long the impact influences the individual. (Source: Livingstone, 2013)

Practitioners can help families to build a familial culture of support so that children can develop digital resilience rather than fearing retribution and punishment, or having their devices confiscated. Children fare better when they believe they will be supported by parents and can go to the parents when upset or distressed about online issues, than those who believe they need to keep their online behaviour and interests invisible from their parents (Livingstone & Blum-Ross, 2020). We advocate working together with families to find ways of recognising that their children are living in a digital age and propose that exclusion is not necessarily always the most appropriate form of protection, but it can be detrimental to their wellbeing and education. It is important that children develop digital resilience to cope with modern adversity.

> **Digital Resilience**
> Refers to the child's ability to positively manage the challenges and negative aspects associated with engaging with others in an online environment.

Thus, it is about helping the child develop digital resilience, learning and adapting in a digital world, recognising the positive from negative influences on them, and having a supportive infrastructure around them when they do find things distressing. More practical support for practitioners can be found in O'Reilly et al. (2021).

Safeguarding

The Oxford English Dictionary definition of the term safeguarding is "to protect from harm or damage with appropriate measure". In its broadest sense would include harm to self as well as harm from others. However, we make a differentiation between harm to self as being something that would be typically treated through the mental health system (albeit within a legal framework), whereas safeguarding in relation to harm from others would usually be managed through social services and justice system. For practitioners, in relation to instructing families about the limits of confidentiality, the risk of immediate harm to self, to others and from others would constitute grounds for legitimately breaching that right. In the context of working with families, we focus here on the aspect of safeguarding as a specific practice-based concern for managing risk of harm from others.

Child Protection

There is a universal concern about the welfare and protection of children from harm and neglect. Many countries have legislation to protect the interests and wellbeing of children. For example, the Department for Education (DfE) in England set out policy, legislation, and statutory guidance for child protection, with the Children Act of 1989 and 2004 providing the legislative framework (NSPCC, 2021a). Similarly, New Zealand has a Children's Act (2014) that prescribes the legal parameters for safeguarding practices. These Acts are designed to offer a structured approach to facilitate collaborative working between agencies to protect and promote the welfare of children and to provide guidance on identifying and supporting children at risk from harm (NSPCC, 2021a). A benefit arising from such legislation was that there is an onus on all organisations working or having contact with children to have safeguarding policies and procedures (NSPCC, 2021b).

Working with families as a practitioner, you are highly likely to engage with children and young people. It is therefore vital that you familiarise yourself with the specific safeguarding policies and procedures of the organisation you work for. Indeed, at the outset of your appointment with an organisation, this should be a priority and usually organisations include safeguarding through induction. For many practitioners, safeguarding training is a mandatory aspect of induction. While these will reflect national legislation, the specific local practices and the named safeguarding contact within the organisation will be different.

Vulnerable Adults

Children are conceptualised as vulnerable by virtue of their status as a minor and their developmental competence. Although the notion of vulnerability is fluid and contested even for children, it is nonetheless a legal reference point that some adult members of society are vulnerable due to reduced capacity or frailty. As noted by Nickel (2006, p. 247):

> Ordinarily, we expect people to safeguard their own rational interests. Some people, however, cannot do this adequately; because of this, their rational interests must be safeguarded institutionally and procedurally.

While safeguarding is an institutional responsibility, its outworking in practice is a procedural matter. There are guiding principles that are useful for practitioners which were offered by NHS England (2014):

- *Empowerment*: Support in decision making and informed consent.
- *Prevention*: Effort to act prior to the occurrence of harm.
- *Proportionality*: Managing risk in the least intrusive manner.
- *Protection:* Advocacy and representation for the most vulnerable.
- *Partnership*: Professional services and community agencies working collaboratively to prevent, detect, and report neglect and abuse.
- *Accountability*: Transparent accountable practices around safeguarding procedures.

Even if certain members of the family are not present in the current interaction, attentiveness to any indications of risk of harm to them from others that the family may mention may require action. For example, they may talk about elderly relatives in a care home or a family member with learning disabilities living in residential care. Additionally, younger members of the family may have taken up roles of caring for other family members. Sometimes the term 'parentified child' is used (especially in family therapy) to describe children who are given or take up age-inappropriate roles and responsibilities with respect to the other children, or in becoming a 'support' to a parent.

Confidentiality Breach

If a potential safeguarding matter is raised while you are working with a family, then there is a probability that you will need to breach confidentiality. In other words, you have duty of care to protect vulnerable persons by reporting concerns that they may have that a person may be at immediate risk of harm from others. From the perspective of informed consent, it is important to have previously discussed with the family the boundaries of the confidentiality agreement you have with them, so that there is a foundational dialogue and shared understanding of the conditions within which a confidentiality breach might need to occur.

It is typically accepted that people have the right to privacy and confidentiality of information about their mental health (Royal College of Psychiatrists, 2017). However, there are a limited number of exceptions to this expectation. Confidentiality is not absolute (General Medical Council [GMC], 2017). The basis for breaching confidentiality is the premise that the protection of the public interest supersedes the rights to privacy of information for the individual (GMC, 2017; NHS, 2003). Typically, the family practitioner only needs to report concerns about potential safeguarding matters to the relevant authorities who will then take responsibility for further investigation.

If a safeguarding concern arises, it is good practice to alert the family to the fact that other agencies will be contacted. This is a lot easier if the practitioner has already outlined the procedure of breach from the outset of the first appointment with that family. We provide a good example of a practitioner (Community Psychiatric Nurse [CPN]) outlining to a child during an initial mental health assessment, the parameters of the confidentiality agreement and the specific circumstances under which the nurse would be obliged to take further action.

Family 21 (from previously unpublished data)

```
CPN    (.hhh) what we speak about is confidential (.) okay
       (0.95)
       the only time that that would get broken (.) would be:
       <if you told me that> (0.82) you'd got thoughts of
       hurting your↓self or hurting other people (0.49) or that
```

```
(.) somebody was hurting ↓you
(0.30)
okay then we'd have to sort of inform somebody ↓else but
otherwise it kind of (0.32) just stays with us
```

This extract succinctly demonstrates the basic protocol of explaining the three exceptions to the confidentiality agreement *'hurting yourself', 'hurting other people',* or *'somebody was hurting you'*. Although in this extract the child does not verbally express understanding these exceptions, the pauses indicate space for the child to acknowledge what is being said. The fact that the CPN continues indicates implicitly if not explicitly (the child may have expressed nonverbally off camera) that the child has agreed to the conditions outlined. However, while this is a clear and simple example of how to introduce the limits of confidentiality to family members, it is often the case that practitioners omit to fully explain these boundaries. The next extract is an example of a partial confidentiality discussion (also from an initial mental health assessment).

Family 28 (from previously unpublished data)

```
Doctor    Okay an:d it's confidential we will not break that
          confidentiality unless we absolutely have to
          (1.37)
          Okay
Child     Uh huh
Doctor    Alright
```

This extract shows that the confidentiality conversation has been raised and that there may be times when the confidentiality might need to be breached *'unless we absolutely have to'*. However, the limitations of this example are that the exact parameters of the circumstances in which this might need to happen are left ambiguous.

> It is very important to outline the limitations of confidentiality with the three specific exceptions: harm to self, others and from others.

Responsibility and Boundaries

Although explaining the limitations of the confidentiality agreement is vitally important for protecting the safety of the family members and others in the community, the burden of protecting confidentiality on the practitioner means it is not ethically or professionally appropriate for them to speak about client matters to anyone apart from a few specific exceptions. In line with the usual principles of managing these exceptions, guidelines usually refer to who needs to know and to only sharing the most limited information. Those exceptions would usually be specific colleagues and/or clinical supervisors. The following extract is taken from our LOSST LIFFE project on professional perspectives of working with suicidal persons. This is a narrative from a private counsellor in the UK who participated in a qualitative interview about their work.

```
I've got a lovely, supportive family but there's obviously the
confidentiality side of things, you know, meaning that I can't
discuss very much when I come home... So, my main source is,
um, would be like peer support, clinical supervision and, um,
trying to do some nice family (activities)
```

(Participant two, private counsellor)

It is standard practice for counsellors, psychologists, psychotherapists, and so forth to have clinical supervision which provides a forum for discussing cases and to debrief about the emotional impact on the practitioner. Additionally, many allied health professionals also engage regularly in clinical supervision. We regard this as best practice. However, some family practitioners such as those in social care, probation, policing, or nursing may not have access to clinical supervision as standard practice. It may be part of the culture of that specific profession to 'just get on with the job' and not take time to reflect on the personal or emotional impact of the work, and yet our work on the LOSST LIFFE project shows very clearly that working with risk can have an emotional impact (see Thorne and O'Reilly, 2022). We therefore encourage you to undertake the reflective activity in Box 9.3.

> **Box 9.3 Reflecting on the Personal Impact of Working with Risk**
>
> Reflective activity
>   Working with risk
>   It is important to be mindful that whatever professional role you are in, you are still human, and it is inevitable when working with families, especially where risk areas are disclosed, that some of the things you encounter will have an emotional resonance. Using avoidance or detachment strategies to suppress your emotional response to having conversations with families about risk can lead to burnout, compassion fatigue, vicarious trauma, and other mental and physical health difficulties.
>   Consider the following list of strategies that you could engage in to build your own resilience and maintain your professional capacity to work effectively with risk in the family:
>
> - Seek out professional supervision on a regular basis for debriefing and planning for proactive coping strategies.
> - Schedule space in the diary for reflection and processing.
> - Take a mindful approach to your work with families by engaging in micro-strategies throughout the day, such as breathing exercises, being present, and connecting with the environment in a sensory way.
> - Find professional colleagues with whom you can safely talk about a family's issues within the boundaries of confidentiality.
> - Make a list of activities that you find relaxing and can help you take your mind off work-related concerns.
> - Find out what wellbeing supports your organisation offers.

Final Thoughts

In this chapter, we have outlined the three main domains of risk and provided data extracts from our research projects to illustrate ways in which practitioners can introduce and discuss these topics in conversations with families. Although there might be reasons why conversations about risk are avoided or overlooked, we have discussed the ways in which not only are these conversations important but have also provided some clear guidelines about how to have those conversations. We now turn to the voice of Alison Drewett who reflects on the issues raised in this chapter in Box 9.4.

Box 9.4 Practitioner Voice, Alison Drewett

Practitioner voices
Alison Drewett
Speech and language therapist

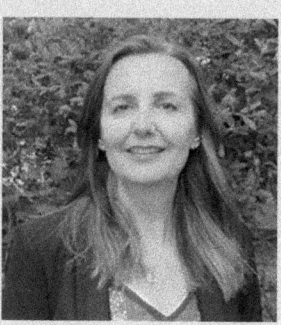

Alison Drewett is a researcher at Loughborough University and is a Highly Specialist Speech and Language Therapist at Leicestershire Partnership (NHS) Trust. She is also studying for her PhD at the University of Leicester around autism and mental health.

My role as a speech and language therapist working in inpatient mental health settings often involved conversations around risk and always necessitated knowing about risk. Staff are specifically mandated to know about patient risk and to plan care accordingly. I quickly learned, as a new professional, that I always needed to talk to the patient's staffing team *before* visiting a patient. I needed to know about the patient's current observation levels, their level of family contact, and their specific risks to plan my therapy sessions accordingly. For example, patients may be care planned to always have a member of staff with them in addition to the therapy staff, or they may have had difficult home leave experiences affecting their mental health or be prevented from carer visits, making references to family sensitive. In addition, they may not be allowed to go off the ward or to have specific objects because of particular identified risks. This would mean that carrying out a social skills session with the person that provided opportunities for interacting with wider members of the community outside the ward environment was not feasible. These examples underline how knowing about risk, understanding family dynamics, and adjusting for risks, is inherent in the clinician's practice. It is core business, not simply a healthcare task.

(*continued*)

Box 9.4 (continued)

Progressing a patient through hospital to discharge inevitably involves many decisions about risk to ensure patient safety and needs family involvement. As well as risk being core business it is also everyone's business, not just the realm of the psychiatrist, clinical psychologist, named nurse or management. For example, it is the responsibility of all staff to ensure that record-keeping is accurate and reporting procedures are followed to guarantee that current information is properly relayed and acted upon. This is essential as risk is dynamic; its patterning can change quickly, especially in acute mental health where the patient is very unwell when admitted, and there is a critical time of getting to know the person, gathering often fragmented and conflicting historical data, and establishing baselines. I have seen serious failures when information about a patient has not been communicated effectively within a team, and the emergence of risky behaviours has not been acted upon and managed. Risk assessment is key to good care, but this also requires effective reporting procedures, as well as frontline staff and families to feel empowered to input into these processes.

During discharge from an inpatient unit for example, a key issue is to talk about is risk. The family play an important role in managing risk in the community, and so, the transition from inpatient care to the community is pivotal. To ensure effective risk management, it is important that families are involved in discharge conversations.

From our experience of clinical practice, research, and supervising and training others, we acknowledge that talking about risk and managing the safeguarding that arise from those conversations is difficult on several levels. It can be difficult at times to initiate those conversations with families, it can be difficult to navigate conversations to identify risk factors, it can be difficult to have to engage agencies to protect family members from harm, and it can be difficult to manage your own emotional responses to risk scenarios. However, the overriding concern is to always think about the wellbeing and safety of family members and the surrounding community which is the motivating factor to ensure these risk procedures are always engaged. Furthermore, we always endeavour to practice what we preach by engaging in self-care strategies because of the type of work in which we are involved. We summarise the key messages from the chapter in Box 9.5.

Box 9.5 Key Points

- There are three areas of risk to assess for in families, harm to self, harm to others, and harm from others.
- Sometimes family members may be at risk of harm to others and from others.
- Asking questions about risk is necessary and there are different styles of questioning that can be useful, such as incremental and normalising.
- Not all risk occurs in the physical environment, so it is helpful to be mindful of family members' digital activity.
- It is essential to outline the limits of confidentiality.
- Safeguarding concerns must be reported to appropriate agencies.
- Working with risk requires additional care to be taken in looking after your own welfare.

References

Aseltine, R., James, A., Schilling, E., & Glanovsky, J. (2007). Evaluating the SOS suicide prevention program: A replication and extension. *BMC Public Health, 7*, 161.

Bajaj, P., Borreani, E., Ghosh, P., Methuen, C., Patel, M., & Crawford, M. (2008). Screening for suicidal thoughts in primary care: The views of patients and general practitioners. *Mental Health Family Medicine, 5*, 229–235.

Baker, K. (2010). More harm than good? The language of public protection. *The Howard Journal of Criminal Justice, 49*(1), 42–53.

Barrocas, A., Hankin, B., Young, J., & Abela, J. (2012). Rates of nonsuicidal self-injury in youth: Age, sex, and behavioral methods in a community sample. *Pediatrics, 130*(1), 39–45.

Blakemore, S. (2018). Avoiding social risk in adolescence. *Current Directions in Psychological Science, 27*(2), 116–122.

Bostik, K., & Everall, R. (2006). In my mind I was alone: Suicidal adolescents' perceptions of attachment relationships. *International Journal for the Advancement of Counselling, 28*(3), 269–287.

Dazzi, T., Gribble, R., Wessely, S., & Fear, N. (2014). Does asking about suicide and related behaviours induce suicide ideation? What is the evidence? *Psychological Medicine, 44*, 3361–3363.

Dekel, B., & Andipatin, M. (2016). Abused women's understandings of intimate partner violence and the link to intimate femicide. *Forum Qualitative Sozialforschung/Forum: Qualitative Social Research, 17*(1) online.

General Medical Council. (2017). *Confidentiality: Good practice in handling patient information*. GMC.

Griffin, E., McMahon, E., McNicholas, F., Corcoran, P., Perry, I., & Arensman, E. (2018). Increasing rates of self-harm among children, adolescents and young adults: A 10-year national registry study, 2007-2016. *Social Psychiatry and Psychiatric Epidemiology, 53*(7), 663–671.

Hawton, K., Saunders, K., & O'Connor, R. (2012). Self-harm and suicide in adolescents. *Lancet, 379*, 2373–2382.

Her Majesty's Inspectorate of Probation. (2008). On the right road (risk of harm inquiry report). Her Majesty's Inspectorate of Probation.

Hornor, G. (2005). Domestic violence and children. *Journal of Pediatric Health Care, 19*(4), 206–212.

Kaufman, J., & Henrich, C. (2000). Exposure to violence and early childhood trauma. In C. H. Zeanah (Ed.), *Handbook of infant mental health* (2nd ed., pp. 195–207). The Guilford Press.

Kiyimba, N., & O'Reilly, M. (2018). Reflecting on what 'you said' as a way of reintroducing difficult topics in child mental health assessments. *Child and Adolescent Mental Health, 23*(3), 148–154.

Klonsky, E., Qiu, T., & Saffer, B. (2017). Recent advances in differentiating suicide attempters from suicide ideators. *Current Opinion in Psychiatry, 30*, 15–20.

Livingstone, S. (2013). Online risk, harm, and vulnerability: Reflections on the evidence base for child Internet safety policy. *ZER: Journal of Communication Studies, 18*(35), 13–28.

Livingstone, S., & Blum-Ross, A. (2020). *Parenting for a digital future: How hopes and fears about technology shape children's lives*. Oxford University Press.

Livingstone, S., & Stoilova, M. (2021). *The 4Cs: Classifying online risk to children. (CO:RE Short Report Series on Key Topics)*. Leibniz-Institut für Medienforschung | Hans-Bredow-Institut (HBI); CO:RE—Children Online: Research and Evidence.

Lutenbacher, M., Cohen, A., & Conner, N. (2004). Breaking the cycle of family violence: Understanding the perceptions of battered women. *Journal of Pediatric Health Care, 18*, 236–242.

NHS. (2003). Code of practice: Confidentiality. Retrieved from: https://assets.publishing.service.gov.uk/government/uploads/system/uploads/attachment_data/file/200146/Confidentiality_-_NHS_Code_of_Practice.pdf.

NHS England. (2014). Safeguarding adults. Retrieved from: https://www.england.nhs.uk/wp-content/uploads/2017/02/adult-pocket-guide.pdf.

NHS Digital (2019). Therapy-based outcomes analysis interactives dashboard. Retrieved from: https://digital.nhs.uk/data-andinformation/publications/statistical/psychological-therapies-report-on-the-use-of-iapt-services/february-2019-including-reports-on-the-iapt-pilots

Nickel, P. (2006). Vulnerable populations in research: The case of the seriously ill. *Theoretical Medicine and Bioethics, 27*(3), 245–264.

NSPCC. (2021a). Child protection system in England. Retrieved from: https://learning.nspcc.org.uk/child-protection-system/england.

NSPCC. (2021b). Safeguarding children and child protection. Retrieved from: https://learning.nspcc.org.uk/safeguarding-child-protection.

Office for National Statistics. (2016). Deaths registered in England and Wales (Series DR). Retrieved from: https://www.one.gov.uk/peoplepopulationandcommunity/birthsdeathsandmarriages/deaths/bulletins/deathsregisteredinenglandandwalesseriesdr/2016.

Office for National Statistics. (2020). Domestic abuse victim characteristics, England and Wales: year ending March 2020. Retrieved from https://www.ons.gov.uk/peoplepopulationandcommunity/crimeandjustice/articles/domesticabusevictimcharacteristicsenglandandwales/yearendingmarch2020.

O'Reilly, M. (2008). "I didn't violent punch him": Parental accounts of punishing children with mental health problems. *Journal of Family Therapy., 30*, 272–295.

O'Reilly, M., Dogra, N., Levine, D., and Donoso, V. (2021). Digital media and child and adolescent mental health: A practical guide to understanding the evidence. .

O'Reilly, M., & Kiyimba, N. (2019). "They nearly got me battered": Self-defence accounts for children's violence. *Conversation analysis of clinical encounters (CACE) international conference, July 2019.* Bristol, UK.

O'Reilly, M., Kiyimba, N., & Karim, K. (2016). "This is a question we have to ask everyone": Asking young people about self-harm and suicide. *Journal of Psychiatric and Mental Health Nursing, 23*, 479–488.

O'Reilly, M., & Parker, N. (2014). 'She needs a smack in the gob': Negotiating what is appropriate talk in front of children in family therapy. *Journal of Family Therapy, 36*(3), 287–307.

Oxford English Dictionary (2018). *Oxford English dictionary online version.* https://en.oxforddictionaries.com/definition/resilience.

Piotrowski, N., & Hartmann, P. (2019). *Magill's medical guide.* Salem Press.

Plaisted, K. C., & Sahakian, B. J. (1997). Dementia of frontal lobe type-living in the here and now. *Aging & Mental Health, 1*(4), 293–295.

Royal College of Psychiatrists. (2017). Good psychiatric practice: Confidentiality and information sharing: third edition. Retrieved from: https://www.rcpsych.ac.uk/docs/default-source/improving-care/better-mh-policy/college-reports/college-report-cr209.pdf?sfvrsn=23858153_2.

Steinberg, L. (2010). A dual systems model of adolescent risk-taking. *Developmental Psychobiology, 52*, 216–224.

The Children's Act. (2014). Oranga Tamariki—Ministry for Children and the Ministry of Education. New Zealand. Retrieved from: https://www.legislation.govt.nz/act/public/2014/0040/latest/whole.html.

Thorne, B., & O'Reilly, M. (2022). Operationalizing strategic objectives of suicide prevention policy: Police-led LOSST LIFFE model. *Death Studies, 46*(9), 2077–2084.

World Health Organization. (2019). *Suicide in the world: Global Health estimates.* WHO.

World Health Organization. (2014). *Preventing suicide: A global imperative.* WHO.

Zeman, J., Cassano, M., Perry-Parrish, C., & Stegall, S. (2006). Emotional regulation in children and adolescents. *Journal of Developmental and Behavioral Pediatrics, 27*(2), 155–168.

10

Using Naturally Occurring Data for Professional Development

Learning Objectives

- Define naturally occurring data
- Recognise the value of recording actual conversations with families for professional development
- Identify some ways that naturally occurring recordings and transcripts can be used for reflective practice and supervision
- Critically assess the potential value of interventionist conversation analysis for supporting professional development

Introduction

In our opening chapter, we introduced you to the concept of naturally occurring data in the context of our research projects that have served as a foundation of examples throughout this book. As a reminder, these are data that capture naturally occurring activities or texts for research purpose as compared with retrospective accounts such as those produced by interviews or focus groups (Kiyimba et al., 2019). The problem with researcher-generated data from interviews and focus groups is that the narratives are subject to a range of biases, such as inaccuracies of memory or deliberate omissions or embellishments. Much therapy research as well as therapy training materials focus on these kinds of accounts, often via post-session checklists and questionnaires or more in-depth post-session interviews. By demonstrating the points raised in the book so far with extracts of in situ conversations with families, we have sought to exemplify the value of using actual naturally occurring transcripts of conversations to study the practices of conversing with families. We acknowledge the caveat that of course, this hinges on how the transcript or video recording captures the process without undue influence imposed by the presence of a recording device. Similarly, in a professional setting, when people talk about interactions and conversations they have had with families, there is the potential for distortion from what actually happened. Therefore, this chapter invites a discussion about the benefits of using actual recordings or written documents that occur naturally in the professional context as a starting point for professional development.

Using Recordings of Naturally Occurring Activities

For some professions it is not unusual to record mental health conversations with families for a variety of reasons, like supervision, training, reflecting teams, and research projects, whilst for other professions it is rarely or never done. However, with an increase in the use of digital and online modalities for working with families and colleagues, these afford more opportunities for recording conversations.

Pragmatics of Recording Conversations with Families

The first consideration when planning to record conversations with families is that of consent. Obviously, covert recording of conversations would be unethical and ensuring that all parties are aware of and have consented to being recorded is essential. There are a range of ways of taking consent from all parties, including asking them to sign a form, all parties verbally expressing their consent for the recording, or in advance notification of the recording taking place and by attending, they are consenting. This is different in the research context which has a more formal governance process, and some organisations also have more official policies or strategies around the taking of consent for professional development purposes. Where there are children involved, the usual protocol is to ask the adult parents or carers to consent on their behalf, however children themselves can also be asked for assent and this is good practice. For families to make an informed decision about consenting to a recording they need to be provided with information about what the recording will be used for, who will have access to it, where it will be stored, and for how long.

After ethical considerations have been accounted for, the next issue in terms of the pragmatics of recording to plan is how to ensure that the recording quality is good so that it is easy to hear what people are saying when creating a transcript. One of the most frustrating things is to have high-quality data but a poor-quality recording so that some of the data is lost or potentially misrepresented. Even if the recording is not transcribed, difficulty in seeing or hearing what people are doing or saying can mean that the value of recording the conversation is significantly diminished. For example, if the recording is being used for supervision purposes, but only the family member is audible and the practitioner's voice cannot be heard because of the location of the recording device, it is impossible for the supervisor to assess the input of the practitioner.

We also offer a caution to be mindful that the nature of the device you are recording on and the type of storage it offers (e.g., hard drive or cloud), has implications for the safety of the data storage. For example, this can raise questions about the potential ownership of recorded material by platform providers. Additionally, care needs to be taken with shared devices or shared storage spaces that they are not accessible by unauthorised persons. Importantly, there are many regulations, legalities, policies, and so forth that govern data collection and storage, even if that is simply for professional development purposes, and we strongly advise you to familiarise yourself with those that relate to your country, organisation, and profession.

Using Online Modalities

These considerations are particularly pertinent when using online mediums for professional conversations with families. Many professions now use a hybrid of face-to-face and online interactions with clients, and some are completely online. Many publicly available platforms (e.g., Skype, Zoom, Teams) are widely used and in some professions, specialist e-health, m-health, or telehealth platforms have been developed. The reasons why some organisations prefer to use these specialist platforms is because of the possibility of added security, which is important for those that also contain information about clients' personal details. These e-health and m-health platforms are used by a range of mental health professionals in modern practice, and there are currently several training courses available for adapting work to an online environment. It is not our aim at this point to discuss the various pros and cons of in-vivo work with families compared to video-mediated professional interactions. However, we note, from the point of view of the pragmatics of recording sessions, that one of the advantages of video-mediated online platforms is that they can be recorded easily with relatively good quality audio and visual (depending on the device). There are two central benefits to making a recording of an online interaction; first is the possible benefit to the client to have a copy to listen to or watch again later, and second, these recordings can be helpful in the professional development of the practitioner.

The therapeutic benefits of clients having access to a recording of their mental health session are becoming more appreciated, as they can revisit the techniques or strategies, or important points in between sessions. Typically, the practitioner will be the host of the session and is therefore the person who has access to the recording and will then take responsibility for the transfer of the recording if all members agree it is beneficial. On a cautionary note, sharing a recording via email or the cloud might compromise its security in addition to the possibility of other people being able to access it on the family member's device. We recommend that if practitioners wish to engage in this practice, they think carefully about the possible security implications and seek out some specialist advice first. Easily attainable recordings of online or computer-mediated

10 Using Naturally Occurring Data for Professional Development

conversations with families provide the practitioner with opportunities to use these recordings for professional development, supervision, and training purposes.

> Make sure the families have consented to recording the session and are clear about what you are going to use the recording for before undertaking this activity.

In the Clinic Versus on the Go

For some professions, meeting with families in a clinic or inpatient facility means that potentially data can be recorded more easily, especially if there is already audio-visual equipment set up in a purpose-built room (such as family therapy settings). For other practitioners, meeting with family members tends to occur in the community or in the family home. The variability of community settings means that there are more things to consider when attempting to record conversations for professional development purposes:

- Background noise—pets, television/radio, extraneous noises like neighbours revving a car loudly or playing music. In such cases, it is wise to consider how much background noise might be picked up by the recording device or microphone. Some microphones filter out background noise and this may be worth the investment.
- Interruptions—unexpected interruptions from someone knocking on the door, visitors arriving, other members of the household may walk into the room, telephone ringing, and so forth. Where possible it may be helpful to collaborate with family members to consider ways to minimise this challenge.
- Third parties—when ethical procedures have been followed to ensure family members being recorded have given consent, it can be problematic if third parties enter the room after this process has been com-

pleted. If the conversation and recording are in mid flow, it can be difficult to stop and ask for consent for those additional third parties. This could be rectified by asking for retrospective consent after the conversation is completed, or the recording will have to be stopped at the point the third party enters.
- Device location—in community or home settings, it can be challenging to figure out where to locate the recording device, and if using video, a portable tripod may need to be set up. If family members or practitioners are moving about in the course of their professional duties, they may move away from the recording device at certain points potentially interrupting the quality of the recording. Some of these challenges may not be resolvable unless one invests in movable devices such as tie-mics or bodycams.

Asking the Family to Record Events in the Home Environment

One of the challenges for practitioners working with families is that we are not with them every day. So, there may be many instances of the problem behaviour for which they have sought professional help that occur in the home where we are unable to see and hear what is happening. With the exception of professionals who may be called into the home at a time of emergency in the family, very many family practitioners see the family members in an institutional context such as a clinic. Practitioners then rely on what occurs between family members during those institutional interactions, and what the family reports as having happened in the home setting. As we showed in the following extract that was introduced in Chap. 7 (taken from Parker, 2003, p. 138), the adolescent male in this interaction with a family therapist complained that the way his parents behaved towards him at home was quite different from how they presented to the therapist in the session.

10 Using Naturally Occurring Data for Professional Development

Gallagher House

```
Client:     You don't see how they treat me.
            (2)
Client:     Js- nasty really nasty.
            (1.2)
Client:     How they can just (1.6) s- swear at me and, (1)
            threaten to kick my head in an-, (1.4) and [then just
            be as nice as- nice as ↑ pie, =
Therapist:                                              [(I've not
            seen that today)
Client:     = to my sisters.
```

Thus, for the practitioner, a web of different narratives from different family members can feel difficult to untangle. One option that some practitioners use is to ask family members to record instances of the problem as it occurs at home, so that they can bring the recording to show to the therapist (O'Hanlon & Rifkin, 2013). Notably, although this technique may provide valuable information for the practitioner to discuss with the family, it is potentially fraught with ethical challenges. Not least, it is unlikely that the person being recorded engaging in inappropriate or problematic behaviour would stop to concede consent for the recording, nor might the person intending to make a recording stop to ask for consent. Nevertheless, we mention the approach here by way of example of another possible way that naturally occurring data could be used therapeutically in working with families.

Using Naturally Occurring Text-Based Documents

It is not always preferable and/or practical to audio-video record conversations with families for professional development or supervision purposes. While we reiterate the value of using actual naturally occurring recordings of conversations for reflection and personal development, we recognise that in the reality of professional practice, some of the challenges outlined previously may prohibit collection of this kind of information. Another form of naturally occurring information that can be very valuable to review, as an individual practitioner, team, or with a clinical supervisor or mentor, is text-based documents. Although there are lots of types of documentation that could be utilised for these purposes, we focus here on the three main document categories, which are clinical notes, referral documents, and progress and outcome reports.

Clinical Notes

One of the most discussed areas of professional practice is how to write good clinical notes. There are many factors that different professional groups prioritise in terms of what kind of information is valuable or necessary to record, as well as where the notes will be kept, that is, paper files or electronically. For individual practitioners, clinical notes may contain information about risk, about the content of that interaction with the family, and about the goals or actions arising from the session. For individual practitioners, the notes will be designed solely for their own record, whereas notes that are accessible to others, such as in multi-disciplinary teams, the notes may be designed to communicate information to others as well as serve the purpose of recording the information for the practitioner who created them. Another factor that practitioners often need to consider is whether the client themselves may at some point request to see their notes and the possibility of whether the notes may be subpoenaed by a court for legal purposes. These considerations will also impact the way the practitioner writes the notes and the content thereof. It can be really helpful for trainees and newly qualified practitioners to work with a supervisor, mentor, or trainer, in developing their own note-keeping practices, to look at actual examples.

Referral Documents

Referral documents are notoriously scant in content. Anecdotally, this can sometimes be a source of frustration for practitioners involved in triage especially, as it can be difficult to identify which services would be most appropriate based on the information provided. One way that a review of referral documents might be beneficial could be in designing a new referral template. If the information provided in the current format does not sufficiently support a high-quality triage process, one solution might be to reorganise the referral template so that headings are created that request specific information. Alternatively, the referrer may have their own documents that they use but only provide minimal information. If practitioners regularly receive referrals from a particular referrer, then a referral document review may highlight particular trends that can be raised with the referrer to support a more satisfactory process.

Progress and Outcome Reports

A valuable part of the professional interaction between referrers and service providers in family support is that service providers communicate well with referrers by giving progress or outcome reports about the interventions. Good quality, effective, and useful progress and outcome reports are succinct and clear and contain all the relevant information. Again, the skill in writing reports that meet these criteria is one that practitioners need to develop during their training and hone their skills throughout their professional career. Examination of examples of good report writing can therefore be extremely valuable for practitioners developing these skills. The ability to see actual examples rather than just understand the principles can genuinely support skill development.

Using Naturally Occurring Data for Supervision

Supervision can be delivered in different forms, including individual reflective or peer discussions or might involve more hierarchical conversations with a mentor or manager (Helps, 2021). As previously mentioned, not all professional groups have clinical supervision. However, practitioners, such as counsellors, psychologists, and psychotherapists, are required by their professional bodies to engage in supervision with a more senior practitioner. The aim of supervision includes several factors, such as mentoring in a particular therapeutic modality and providing opportunity for reflection on one's own practice (Fruggeri, 2002). The goal of the supervisory process is to support and enhance the skills of the practitioner. This is illustrated below:

> *First, supervision is a central form of support where we can focus on our own difficulties as a worker, as well as have our supervisor share some of the responsibility for our work with the client. Second, supervision forms part of our continual development as workers, including eventually helping us to learn how to be supervisors.*
> (Hawkins & Shohet, 2000, p. 23)

Typically, during supervision, the supervisee will report on their intervention with a family using a retrospective account of their interaction. The value of this is that the supervisee can quickly report on areas that they wish to elicit the advice or guidance of their supervisor, such as when they are feeling 'stuck' with how to progress with a family or when there are complexities relating to risk or safeguarding that the supervisee would like support with. However, all retrospective accounts are subject to deliberate or inadvertent distortion and so bringing in audio, video, or text-based naturally occurring documents to supervision can provide a tangible and concrete basis for discussions about practitioner developments (Helps, 2021).

In the case of video or audio recordings of interactions with families, these can be replayed during supervision for real-time reflection and review. This is often the preferred way to use naturally occurring materials in supervision. However, in the case of trainee practitioners, a more rigorous approach is usually taken which involves producing a written transcript of an audio or visual recording. Although there are now some automated programmes that create simple transcripts such as in Zoom, where these are not available, the creation of a transcript is a more time-consuming process and is the main reason why this approach is often not used beyond the requirement of training programmes. The value of a written transcript, however, is that a more rigorous analysis can be conducted on the nuances of how particular interactional skills are used by the trainee practitioner.

There are also a growing number of commercial databases of anonymised therapeutic interactions with individuals and families that can be used as a training resource. They provide the opportunity to "compare therapeutic methods, relate them back to client outcomes, examine language patterns across different types of psychotherapy, and explore countless other lines of inquiry" (Alexander-Street, 2022, n.p). An advantage of using a pre-existing dataset is that no additional consent or recordings are needed, and the datasets often cover a wide range of topics and therapeutic approaches. However, there is still huge value in trainees and qualified practitioners recording their own work for personal reflection or supervision. It is often the only way that tutors or supervisors can actually see what the trainee is doing in practice (see, e.g., Gale et al., 1993).

Whether the actual audio-visual recording is used in supervision or a transcript, or if both are used simultaneously, the following guidance can provide a helpful framework to engage with naturally occurring examples of practice as recommended by Helps (2021):

1. Prior to your supervision session, it can be helpful to find specific parts of the recording that you are interested in discussing. This may be something that went well or an instance where the supervisee would like some advice on how they may have done things differently.
2. During the supervision, it is useful to discuss with the supervisor things that were noticed about the way in which the conversation proceeded.
3. Discuss with your supervisor things that you have noticed about your communication. Engage with the questions your supervisor raises about the things you noticed to deepen your reflection.
4. Pay particular attention to any discrepancies between your memories of what happened in the client session compared to what can be seen to have genuinely happened using the recording.
5. With your supervisor, create a plan for what you will do differently in future based on your observations and reflections.
6. Discuss how these new understandings and insights might inform the wider context of your work with other families.

An example of how this process might be valuable to reflect on one's own professional practice is demonstrated in the following extracts. Both extracts show how the practitioners ask several questions in the same sentence. The fact that the child in both examples is unable to answer the multiple questions can be seen clearly when a transcript is used for reflective practice and professional development. By looking carefully at these transcripts, the practitioner and their supervisor may be able to construct an alternative way of formulating their enquiry that is clearer and more concise. We provide two examples of previously unpublished data to illustrate.

Family 4

```
OT      ↓an' what things did you enjoy doing to↓gether when you
        were little? What can you re↓member? You look like you
        ↓like mega ↓blocks
        (0.65)
        ↓did you like mega blocks ↓when you were little?
Child   °↑uh°
```

Family 14

```
MHN     So tell me a little bit about when you were coming
        here to↓day (.) What were yo:u hoping for (0.52) eh to
        be different?
        (.)
        What do you think are: the probl↑ems if there are any?
        An' what do you (0.31) want help with?
Child   °(I dunno)°
```

Following our identification of the multiple question problem that some of the practitioners in this set of recordings were facing, we decided to look at a larger set of transcripts to explore whether multiple question asking was a common problem. This led to a wider investigation of question use in initial assessments. By taking a combination of conversation analysis to identify different kinds of questions, and content analysis to ascertain frequencies, we found that across the 28 assessments, a total of 9086 questions were asked to families by practitioners (O'Reilly et al., 2015). This was an average of 323.9 questions per assessment. Across the data were 5327 questions directed towards children and 3714 towards parents, with others having no speaker selection. Thus, the mean number of questions was 3.7 per minute, which is one question approximately every 15 seconds.

During a professional development workshop, the practitioners involved in this study were able to compare the facts that were established by analysis of actual recordings and transcripts, against their subjective retrospective memories. First, they were surprised at the discrepancy between their own subjective experience of how many questions they thought they had asked and the facts established by counting them on the recordings. This demonstrates that the use of recordings can be extremely valuable in identify actual practice versus perceived practice. Second, the practitioners were able to reflect on and discuss the types of questions used, their efficacy, and the way in which they were constructed. Finally, the psychiatrist in the team selected extracts of video to discuss with his own trainees (both those trainees present in the recordings and those not directly involved). Using real-world video recordings of practice (either their own or someone else's) provided a useful mechanism for training and reflection. Evidently, shining a spotlight on your own practice, and the practice of others, which may feel a bit uncomfortable, can be extremely beneficial to you and your peers for continuing professional development.

Using Reflective Interventionist Conversation Analysis (RICA)

In the previous section, we discussed the benefits of watching audio-visual recordings of actual sessions with family members during supervision to facilitate reflective practice and develop professional skills. We also demonstrated some of the benefits of a closer analysis of transcripts of those recordings to highlight patterns and enable critical reflection on certain aspects of practice such as asking questions. In Chap. 9, we demonstrated the value of using conversation analysis as an analytic approach to investigating transcripts and highlighted how this methodology helped the practitioners involved to improve their risk assessment practices. The type of applied conversation analysis that is used specifically to reflect on practice using transcripts of naturally occurring conversations with families is called 'Reflective Interventionist Conversation Analysis [RICA]' (O'Reilly et al., 2020a).

There are several different approaches to applied conversation analysis (CA) (Antaki, 2011), one of which is interventionist CA. A characteristic of interventionist CA is that it is an approach that has the goal of changing aspects of the participants' conduct (Wilkinson, 2014). However, what is unique about RICA as a form of interventionist CA, is that it takes an inductive or unmotivated looking approach to examining transcripts rather than being driven by a previously identified problem (O'Reilly et al., 2020b). The features of interventionist CA are that participants whose voices are represented in the transcript work together in partnership with another person or persons (i.e., a researcher or supervisor), and the implications of those conversations are dually considered (Wilkinson, 2014). The advantage of this for reflective practice and supervision is that good practice examples can be identified as well as considering ways to mitigate identified problems. In the seminal paper on RICA (O'Reilly et al., 2020b), the two potential outcomes were: (1) the identification of good practice, so that practitioners can use these skills more and that supervisors or mentors can utilise core messages as a tool for training or reflection; (2) the identification of areas where change or improvement might be beneficial.

For practitioners interested in using RICA as an empirically informed methodology to examine and reflect on actual professional conversations with families, there are a few considerations to be mindful of. First, because RICA is a form of conversation analysis, there is a conventional approach to transcription, which includes the use of symbols to represent intonation, volume, emphasis, and other paralinguistic features (Jefferson, 2004). There are several resources available, including the original work of Jefferson (2004) and a more recent publication (Hepburn & Bolden, 2017), as well as online tutorials, that can be accessed by practitioners wishing to utilise this method. Second, conversation analysis and RICA in particular are methodologies that require some initial training for the novice user. We encourage you to actively seek out credible internet-based resources and tutorials, as well as training opportunities within your country. Third, we acknowledge that for busy family practitioners, finding the time to invest in this kind of professional development can sometimes be challenging, and it may be necessary to negotiate with your employer for additional time or resources to engage in this form of good practice skill development. Despite these considerations, we highly recommend RICA as an extremely valuable way to review current practice, to reflect on skills and language use, and to engage in dialogue with colleagues to enhance communication with families.

Final Thoughts

We have structured this book into three sections. First, we introduced the theoretical context of communication with families. In this section, we critically examined the way that the family unit is constructed within different cultures and over time and introduced our discursive approach to investigating communication with families. This section also provided tools for managing multi-party interaction with multiple family members. Second, we focused on effective ways to engage with children in professional contexts. This involved an exploration of various discursive and creative strategies to engage children and young people in ways that enable them to feel more comfortable about discussing their feelings and experiences. A discussion of the notion of children's competence was the precursor for critically questioning the appropriateness of children's presence in conversations where certain topics are being discussed. In the final section of this book, we examined the ways in which discursive approaches and conversation analysis can be valuable analytic tools for reflecting upon audio-visual recordings of sessions with family members and transcripts of those recordings for professional development. Specifically, we highlighted the ways in which family members may experience shame and blame and how we might manage that, how risk and self-harm can be discussed safely with family members and how recordings of practice can be used for professional development and supervision. Throughout this book, the practitioner voice boxes have complemented the theory and data that have constituted most of the text for each chapter, by indicating how these concepts might be usefully applied in different professional contexts.

References

Alexander-Street. (2022). *Counseling and psychotherapy transcripts series.* As retrieved from: https://alexanderstreet.com/products/counseling-and-psychotherapy-transcripts-series.

Antaki, C. (2011). Six kinds of applied conversation analysis. In C. Antaki (Ed.), *Applied conversation analysis: Intervention and change in institutional talk* (pp. 1–14). Palgrave Macmillan.

Fruggeri, L. (2002). Different levels of analysis in the supervisory process. In D. Campbell & B. Mason (Eds.), *Perspectives on supervision* (pp. 3–20). Karnac Books.

Gale, J., Dotson, D., Lindsey, E., & Negireddy, C. (1993). Conversation analysis: A method for self-supervision. Paper presented at AAMFT's 51st annual conference, Anaheim, CA.

Hawkins, P., & Shohet, R. (2000). *Supervision in the helping professions* (2nd ed.). Open University Press.

Helps, S. (2021). Developing supra-vision using naturally occurring video material within supervision. In M. O'Reilly & J. N. Lester (Eds.), *Improving communication in mental health settings: Evidence-based recommendations from practitioner-led research.* Routledge.

Hepburn, A., & Bolden, G. (2017). *Transcribing for social research.* Sage.

Jefferson, G. (2004). Glossary of transcript symbols with an introduction. In G. Lerner (Ed.), *Conversation analysis: Studies from the first generation* (pp. 13–31). John Benjamins.

Kiyimba, N., Lester, J., & O'Reilly, M. (2019). *Using naturally occurring data in health research: A practical guide.* Springer.

O'Hanlon, B., & Rifkin, J. (2013). The tape recorder cure. In *Evolving possibilities* (pp. 33–38). Routledge.

O'Reilly, M., Karim, K., & Kiyimba, N. (2015). Question use in child mental health assessments and the challenges of listening to families. *British Journal of Psychiatry Open, 1*(2), 116–120.

O'Reilly, M., Kiyimba, N., Lester, J., & Muskett, T. (2020a). Reflective interventionist conversation analysis. *Discourse & Communication, 14*(6), 619–634.

O'Reilly, M., Muskett, T., Karim, K., & Lester, J. (2020b). Parents' constructions of normality and pathology in child mental health assessments. *Sociology of Health and Illness, 42*(3), 544–564.

Parker, N. (2003). 'What do you think?': A discursive analysis of psychology in therapy talk. Doctoral thesis. Loughborough University.

Wilkinson, R. (2014). Intervening with conversation analysis in speech and language therapy: Improving aphasic conversation. *Research on Language and Social Interaction, 47*(3), 219–238.

Appendix: Jefferson Transcription – Overview of Symbols Used

- (.) A full stop inside brackets denotes a micro pause, a notable pause but of no significant length.
- (0.2) A number inside brackets denotes a timed pause. This is a pause long enough to time and subsequently show in transcription.
- [Square brackets denote a point where overlapping speech occurs.
- > < Arrows surrounding talk like these show that the pace of the speech has quickened.
- < > Arrows in this direction show that the pace of the speech has slowed down.
- ( ) Where there is space between brackets denotes that the words spoken here were too unclear to transcribe.
- (( )) Where double brackets appear with a description inserted denotes some contextual information where no symbol of representation was available.
- **Underline** When a word or part of a word is underlined, it denotes a raise in volume or emphasis.
- ↑ When an upward arrow appears, it means there is a rise in intonation.

- ↓ When a downward arrow appears, it means there is a drop in intonation.
- → An arrow like this denotes a particular sentence of interest to the analyst.
- **CAPITALS** where capital letters appear it denotes that something was said loudly or even shouted.
- **Hum(h)our** When a bracketed 'h' appears it means that there was laughter within the talk.
- = The equal sign represents latched speech, a continuation of talk.
- :: Colons appear to represent elongated speech, a stretched sound.

(Sources: Jefferson, 2004; Hepburn and Bolden, 2017).

Index

A

Abuse, 176
Accountability, 91
Accountable, 200
Active listening, 56
Addiction, 205
Adverse childhood events/experiences (ACEs), 43, 222
Adversity, 37
Alcohol or substance misuse, 222
Alignment, 54–61
Appropriate, 176–180
Archetypes, 124–135
Artefacts, 4
Attachments, 38
Attachment theories, 203

B

Binary, 198
Blame, 197
Blaming, 99
Body language, 4
Bowen, M., 11
Bronfenbrenner, U., 11

C

Child-centred ideology, 87
Childhood, 34
Child protection, 240
Children, 177, 184
 competence, 147–170
 development, 147
 engagement, 68
 rights, 87
Circular questions, 108–110
Clinical notes, 260
Closed questions, 89–90
Communication, 3
Competence/competency, 74, 148, 149, 165–167

Competent, 148
Complaint, 60, 178
Confidentiality, 242–243
Consent, 259
Conversation analysis, 18
Courtesy stigma, 202
COVID-19, 44
Creative activities, 117
Creative modalities, 117
Cultures, 175

D

Dallos, R., 16
Declarative questions, 92–93
Deontic reasoning, 150
Derogatory way, 181
Developmental competence, 157
Developmental theories, 147
Diagnoses, 8
Diagnostic manuals, 8
Dialectical balance, 128, 133
Digital age, 239
Digital devices, 238
Digital health, 136
Digital media, 136
Digital revolution, 136
Discontinuity, 65–67
Discourse, 5
Discourse analysis, 18
Discursive analytic approaches, 3
Discursive psychology, 19
Disruption, 63–64
Domestic violence, 220
Drawings, 119

E

Ecological systems theory, 11–12
Education, 34
e-Health, 140
Emotional harm, 182
Emotional literacy, 159
Epigenetics, 39
Epistemic continuum, 158
Epistemic position, 161
Epistemology, 6
Extreme case formulations, 56

F

Family-based psychological interventions, 45
Family-centred stance, 29
Family dynamics, 30
Family resilience, 38
Family systems, 130
  maps, 131
  theory, 12–15
Family tree, 125
4 P, 39

G

Genograms, 131
Good, 198
Good parent, 200–203
Gossiping, 56, 181

H

Half-membership, 75
Harm, 218

I

Identities, 15
Identity management, 33
Inappropriate, 192
Inappropriate language, 177
Inattention, 62–63
Institutional business, 71
Institutional expectations, 155
Institutional interactions, 149
Institutional scripts, 156
Institutional settings, 152–153
Interactional agenda, 77
Interactional competency, 159, 163
Intergenerational multi-party
   conversations, 192
Interruptions, 69–77
Intimate partner, 220
Intimate partner
   violence, 176

J

Jefferson, G., 19

K

Knowledge (K-), 155
Knowledge (K+), 155
Knowledge competency, 168
Knowledge continuum, 159
K+ K- continuum model, 161

L

Labelling, 8–9
Language, 4
Linguistic competence, 157

M

Marginalised, 192
Medicalise, 206
Medical paradigm, 10
Mental health, 3
Mentoring, 261
Metaphor, 121
Miracle question, 102–106
Moral, 199
Multi-party conversations, 70
Mundane, 152

N

Narrative Therapy (NT), 15
Naturally occurring, 16
   activities, 253
   data, 253
Nature, 199
Neglect, 233
Neurodiversity, 148
Normality, 9
Normal/normalising, 148,
   198, 225–226
Normative script, 150

P

Parental determinism, 200
Parent blaming, 203–205
Pathology, 9
Police, 232
Politeness, 74
Power, 5, 70, 184
Professional development, 255
Progress and outcome reports, 261
Protect, 187

Q

Question and answer sequences, 88

R

Rapport, 55
Recipient selection, 165
Recording, 255
Referral documents, 260–261
Reflected speech, 107
Reflexivity, 3
Reported speech, 107
Resilience, 36–44, 239
Resistance, 64, 106
Rights, 35
Risk, 210, 217
  assessment, 228
  from others, 218
  to others, 218
  to self, 218
Risk-taking, 219
Rupture, 61–69

S

Sacks, H., 159
Safeguarding, 187, 228
Scripts, 151, 153, 156
Self-harm, 220
Separation, 180, 191
Shame, 197
Sick, 198
Situated interactional
  competence, 149–158
Social action, 21
Social competence, 74

Social constructionism, 6
Social constructionist, 6
Social ecologies, 38
Social interactional
  competence, 149
Socially constructed, 198
Social norms, 202
Social schema, 75
Social services, 237
Social worker, 237
Sociology of the child, 34–35
Stigma, 7–9
Stigmatisation, 202
Stigmatising labels, 182
Stress bucket, 121
Stress vulnerability model, 41
Strong, T., 128
Subjective knowledge, 168
Subjective Units of Distress
  Scale, 118
Suicide, 220
Supervisor, 260
Symbolic communication, 5
Symbols, 124–135
Systems theory, 38

T

Tag questions, 93–94
Telehealth, 137
Text-based documents, 259–261
Therapeutic relationship, 54–61
Tomm, K., 125, 197
Topic, 175, 183
Training, 254
Transcripts, 254

Transition relevance places
  (TRPs), 70
Turn taking, 69, 159

U

Unmotivated looking, 16
Using Reflective Interventionist
  Conversation Analysis
  (RICA), 265–267

V

Verbal scale, 118
Violence, 219

Virtue signalling, 208–211
Vulnerability, 36–44, 241
Vulnerable adults, 241

W

Wh-prefaced questions, 90–92
Why question, 99
World Health Organization
  (WHO), 136

Y

You said prefaced
  questions, 106–108

GPSR Compliance
The European Union's (EU) General Product Safety Regulation (GPSR) is a set of rules that requires consumer products to be safe and our obligations to ensure this.

If you have any concerns about our products, you can contact us on

ProductSafety@springernature.com

In case Publisher is established outside the EU, the EU authorized representative is:

Springer Nature Customer Service Center GmbH
Europaplatz 3
69115 Heidelberg, Germany

www.ingramcontent.com/pod-product-compliance
Ingram Content Group UK Ltd.
Pitfield, Milton Keynes, MK11 3LW, UK
UKHW022241180226
468167UK00006B/284